The
Guide to Fat Free Foods©

MW00978248

Post Office Box 1151
Alpharetta, Georgia 30239

Table of Contents

These opening pages are left blank on the back for the shopper's personal observations, comments, or dietary information. There are also pages for notes at the end of the book.

Addresses, Phone Numbers

....

....

....

....

....

....

....

....

....

....

....

....

Introduction

This book has been developed to help everyone "take that weight off of your mind." Fat free foods are no substitute for a balanced diet, but can be a great help when preparing your diet. When choosing snacks, the fat free taste is becoming better each month as food manufacturers realize the significance of taste in generating sales.

Also, the quotes at the bottom of each page are designed to give the reader information, encouragement, and hope as they read over all of the listings of fat free foods.

—Editor

Shopping List

....

....

....

....

....

....

....

....

....

....

....

....

Foreword

They who by their labor get their bread,
in an independent state,
who seldom eat and never beg,
can fix or change their fate.

Notes

Definitions on Labels and Abbreviations

Reduced Fat: Means at least 25% less fat than the typical product.

Light: Means at least one-third fewer calories or 50% less fat.

Low Fat: Is an absolute claim of 3 grams of fat, or less, per serving.

Non Fat or Fat Free: Is less than one half gram of fat per serving

Monounsaturated Fats: May reduce your blood cholesterol level. This type of fat is found in olive oil, canola oil, avocados, and certain other plant foods.

Polyunsaturated Fats: Also reduces blood cholesterol levels. This type of fat is found in products made from sunflowers, corn, and soybeans.

Abbreviations

Oz. = Ounce
Fl. Oz. = Fluid Ounce
FF = Fat Free
Fzn. = Frozen
Reg. = Regular
Ml. = Millilitre

Pkt. = Packet
Lb. = Pound
Tbsp. = Tablespoon
FF = Fat Free
Tsp. = Teaspoon

Notes

....

....

....

....

....

....

....

....

....

....

....

Disclaimer

This book is intended as a guide for those people who ish to locate fat free foods. The author expresses an pinion, but does not give advice. This book should not e looked upon as a diet book. It is the intention of the uthor for this book to be used only as a reference guide fat free foods.

Sources of Information/Data

The U.S. Department of Agriculture, Food and utrition Service, Southeast Region, 77 Forsyth Street, W, Atlanta, Georgia 30303.

Information from food labels, manufacturers, and ocessors. Manufacturer's ingredients are subject to ange, so current values may vary from those listed in is book.

A special thank you to Kelloggs, Health Valley, ealthy Choice, Pepperidge Farm, Brach's, Bresler's, 'eight Watchers, Edy's, Royal, Kraft, Dannon, Yoplait, uaker, Welch's, Smuckers, Del Monte, and all of the od manufacturers who provided the information for this ook.

Notes

....

....

....

....

....

....

....

....

....

....

....

The Food Pyramid

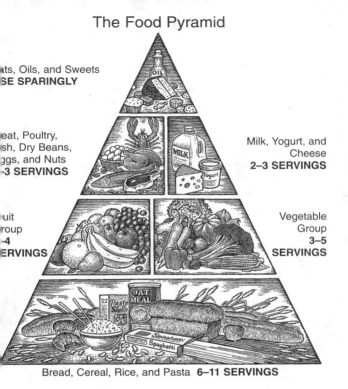

ts, Oils, and Sweets
SE SPARINGLY

eat, Poultry,
sh, Dry Beans,
gs, and Nuts
-3 SERVINGS

Milk, Yogurt, and Cheese
2–3 SERVINGS

uit
roup
-4
ERVINGS

Vegetable Group
3–5
SERVINGS

Bread, Cereal, Rice, and Pasta **6–11 SERVINGS**

he Pyramid is a general guide to help you make your aily nutritional choices.

Notes

....

....

....

....

....

....

....

....

....

....

....

....

Beverages

Product	Manufacturer	Serving Size	Calories
All Natural Grape Drink	Welch's	6 fl. oz.	120
American Lager	Stroh's	12 fl. oz.	145
Apple Citrus	Tree Top	6 fl. oz.	90
Apple-Berry Drink	Juice Works	6 fl. oz.	100
Apple-Cherry Drink	Juice + More	8 fl. oz.	120
Apple-Cranberry Drink	Mott's	6 fl. oz.	83
Apple-Cranberry Drink	Tree Top	6 fl. oz.	100
Apple-Grape Drink	Juice + More	8 fl. oz.	120
Apple-Grape Drink	Juicy Juice	6 fl. oz.	90
Apple-Grape Drink	Mott's	9.5 fl. oz.	139
Apple-Raspberry Drink	Tree Top	6 fl. oz.	80
Apple-Grape-Cherry Drink	Welch's Orchard	6 fl. oz.	100
Apple-Pear Drink	Tree Top	6 fl. oz.	90
Apple-Raspberry Drink	Juice + More	8 fl. oz.	120
Apple-Raspberry Drink	Tree Top	6 fl. oz.	80
b & b	generic	1 fl. oz.	94
Beer	Black Horse	12 fl. oz.	158
Beer	Carlsburg	12 fl. oz.	149
Beer	Heineken	12 fl. oz.	152
Beer	King Cobra	12 fl. oz.	182
Beer	Kronenbourg	12 fl. oz.	170
Beer	Lowenbrau	12 fl. oz.	157

Never go to the grocery store hungry.

Beverages

Product	Manufacturer	Serving Size	Calories
Beer	Michelob	12 fl. oz.	160
Beer	Old Milwaukee	12 fl. oz.	145
Beer	Pilsner	12 fl. oz.	145
Beer, Blue Light	Labatt's	12 fl. oz.	115
Beer, Blue Ribbon	Pabst	12 fl. oz.	144
Beer, Blue Ribbon extra light	Pabst	12 fl. oz.	70
Beer, Bock	Stroh's	12 fl. oz.	157
Beer, Bud Dry	Anheuser-Busch	12 fl. oz.	130
Beer, Bud Light	Anheuser-Busch	12 fl. oz.	110
Beer, Busch Light Draft	Anheuser-Busch	12 fl. oz.	110
Beer, Classic Dark	Michelob	12 fl. oz.	164
Beer, Coor's Light	Coor's	12 fl. oz.	105
Beer, Corona Light	Corona	12 fl. oz.	105
Beer, Dark Special	Lowenbrau	12 fl. oz.	158
Beer, Dry	Coor's	12 fl. oz.	119
Beer, Dry	Keystone	12 fl. oz.	121
Beer, Dry	Michelob	12 fl. oz.	130
Beer, Extra Gold	Coor's	12 fl. oz.	151
Beer, Genuine Draft Light	Miller	12 fl. oz.	98
Beer, High Life	Miller	12 fl. oz.	147
Beer, Light	Amstel	12 fl. oz.	95
Beer, Light	Carlsburg	12 fl. oz.	110
Beer, Light	Keystone	12 fl. oz.	100
Beer, Light	Lowenbrau	12 fl. oz.	98
Beer, Light	Michelob	12 fl. oz.	134
Beer, Light	Molson	12 fl. oz.	109

Always check food product labels to suit your needs.

Beverages

Product	Manufacturer	Serving Size	Calories
Beer, Light	Old Milwaukee	12 fl. oz.	120
Beer, Light	Stroh's	12 fl. oz.	115
Beer, Light	Blatz	12 fl. oz.	96
Beer, Light	generic	12 fl. oz.	95
Beer, Light	generic	12 fl. oz.	100
Beer, Light Amber	New Amsterdam	12 fl. oz.	95
Beer, Lite	Miller	12 fl. oz.	96
Beer, Natural Light	Anheuser-Busch	12 fl. oz.	110
Beer, Non-Alcoholic	Pabst	12 fl. oz.	55
Beer, Non-Alcoholic	Moussy	12 fl. oz.	50
Beer, Original	Coor's	12 fl. oz.	137
Beer, Original	Keystone	12 fl. oz.	121
Beer, Red	Killian's	12 fl. oz.	127
Beer, regular	generic	12 fl. oz.	146
Beer, regular	generic	12 fl. oz.	150
Beer, Reserve Light, 100% Barley Draft	Miller	12 fl. oz.	106
Beer, Special	Lowenbrau	12 fl. oz.	158
Beer, Special Dark	Heineken	12 fl. oz.	192
Bitter Lemon	Schweppe's	6 fl. oz.	78
Black Cherry Cider	Crystal Geyser	6 fl. oz.	60
Black Cherry Drink	Kool-Aid	8 fl. oz.	98
Black Label	Carling	12 fl. oz.	136
Bloody Mary	Libby	6 fl. oz.	40
Brandy	generic	1 fl. oz.	75
Champagne	generic	4 fl. oz.	84
Club Soda	Schweppe's	8 fl.oz.	0
Cocktail, bourbon & soda	generic	4 fl. oz.	105

If you are overweight, consult your lifestyle

Beverages

Product	Manufacturer	Serving Size	Calories
Cocktail, black russian	generic	3 fl. oz.	255
Cocktail, bloody mary	generic	8 fl. oz.	184
Cocktail, daiquiri	generic	3.5 fl. oz.	122
Cocktail, daiquiri	generic	2 fl. oz.	111
Cocktail, gin & tonic	generic	7.5 fl. oz.	171
Cocktail, highball	generic	8 fl. oz.	165
Cocktail, manhattan	generic	1 fl. oz.	27
Cocktail, margarita	generic	1 fl. oz.	4
Cocktail, margarita	generic	3.5 fl. oz.	122
Cocktail, martini	generic	3.5 fl. oz.	140
Cocktail, martini	generic	2.5 fl. oz.	156
Cocktail, mint julep	generic	10 fl. oz.	215
Cocktail, pina colada	generic	4.5 fl. oz.	347
Cocktail, screwdriver	generic	7 fl. oz.	174
Cocktail, sloe gin fizz	generic	8 fl. oz.	121
Cocktail, tequila sunrise	generic	5.5 fl. oz.	189
Cocktail, tom collins	generic	7.5 fl. oz.	121
Coconut Pineapple Nectar	Kern's	6 fl. oz.	120
Coffee, brewed	Espresso	2 fl. oz.	1
Coffee, decaffeinated	Kava	1 tsp.	4
Coffee, decaffeinated	Taster's Choice	6 fl. oz.	4
Coffee, decaffeinated	generic	1 tsp.	0
Coffee, instant	Kava	1 tsp.	2
Coffee, instant	generic	1/4 cup	10
Coffee, regular	Taster's Choice	6 fl. oz.	4
Coffee, regular	Kava	1 tsp.	4
Coffee, regular	generic	6 fl. oz.	0

You have the answers for a healthier life – take control.

Beverages

Cola, diet	generic	12 fl. oz.	0
Cola, regular	generic	12 fl. oz.	160
Collin's Mixer	Schweppe's	6 fl. oz.	70
Cordial/Liqueur	generic	1 fl. oz.	97
Cran-Blueberry	Ocean Spray	6 fl. oz.	120
Cran-Cherry Drink	Ocean Spray	6 fl. oz.	120
Cran-Grape	Ocean Spray	6 fl. oz.	120
Cran-Raspberry	Ocean Spray	6 fl. oz.	110
Cran-Raspberry Low Calorie	Ocean Spray	6 fl. oz.	40
Cran-tastic	Ocean Spray	6 fl. oz.	110
Cranapple	Ocean Spray	6 fl. oz.	120
Cranapple, Low Calorie	Ocean Spray	6 fl. oz.	40
Dark Ale	Becks	12 fl. oz.	156
Diet 7-Up	Dr. Pepper	6 fl. oz.	0
Diet Cherry 7-Up	Dr. Pepper	6 fl. oz.	2
Diet Cherry Coke	Coca-Cola	6 fl. oz.	0
Diet Chocolate Fudge Soda	Canfield's	6 fl. oz.	2
Diet Coke	Coca-Cola	6 fl. oz.	0
Diet Crystal Clear Pepsi	Pepsi Cola	6 fl. oz.	0
Diet Dr. Pepper	Dr. Pepper	6 fl. oz.	0
Diet Minute Maid Soda	Coca-Cola	6 fl. oz.	4
Diet Mountain Dew	Pepsi Cola	6 fl. oz.	2
Diet Orange	Faygo	6 fl. oz.	0
Diet Pepsi Clear	Pepsi Cola	6 fl. oz.	0
Diet Pineapple-Orange	Faygo	6 fl. oz.	0

G.E.N. – Greed Exceeds Need.

Beverages

Product	Manufacturer	Serving Size	Calories
Diet Red Pop	Faygo	6 fl. oz.	0
Diet Root Beer	A & W	6 fl. oz.	0
Diet Root Beer	Faygo	6 fl. oz.	0
Diet Root Beer	I.B.C.	12 fl. oz.	4
Diet Slice	Pepsi Cola	6 fl. oz.	2
Diet Sprite	Coca-Cola	6 fl. oz.	2
Diet Vanilla Soda	A & W	6 fl. oz.	0
Espresso	generic	6 fl. oz.	0
Extra Stout	Guinness	12 fl. oz.	192
Faygo Frosh	Faygo	6 fl. oz.	0
Florida Citrus Punch	Sunny Delight	6 fl. oz.	90
Foster's Light Lager	Foster's	12 fl. oz.	88
Fresca	Coca-Cola	6 fl. oz.	2
Fruit Island Punch Cocktail	Hawaiian Punch	6 fl. oz.	90
Fruit Juicy Red	Hawaiian Punch	6 fl. oz.	90
Fruit Punch	Bama	8.45 fl. oz.	130
Fruit Punch	Mott's	9.5 fl. oz.	150
Fruit Punch	Sipp's	8.45 fl. oz.	130
Fruit Punch	Staff	6 fl. oz.	90
Fruit Punch	Coca-Cola	8 fl. oz.	70
Fruit Punch, canned	Staff	6 fl. oz.	85
Fruit Tea Cooler, as prepared	Lipton	8 fl. oz.	87
Gin, 80% proof	generic	1.5 fl. oz.	95
Gin, 86% proof	generic	1.5 fl. oz.	105
Gin, 90% proof	generic	1.5 fl. oz.	110
Ginger Ale	generic	12 fl. oz.	125
Ginger Ale, diet	Schweppe's	12 fl. oz.	3

You can tell when you eat well, and so can others.

Beverages

Product	Manufacturer	Serving Size	Calories
Ginger Ale, Raspberry	Schweppe's	8 fl. oz.	100
Ginger Ale, Raspberry, diet	Schweppe's	8 fl. oz.	0
Grape Drink	Gatorade	8 fl. oz.	50
Grape Drink, canned	generic	6 fl. oz.	100
Grape Soda	generic	12 fl. oz.	180
Grape-Apple Drink	Mott's	9.5 fl. oz.	158
Hawaiian Guava Fruit Drink	Mauna L'ai	6 fl. oz.	100
Hawaiian Passion Fruit Drink	Mauna L'ai	6 fl. oz.	100
Hawaiian Punch, FF	Sundor Brands	8 fl. oz.	110
Hot Cocoa Mix, diet	Carnation	1 envelope	25
Ice Tea Mix, w/sugar & lemon	Nestle	8 fl. oz.	70
Ice Tea, Crystal Light Sugar Free, Lemon	Kraft	8 fl. oz.	4
Ice Tea, Crystal Light Sugar Free, Pink	Kraft	8 fl. oz.	4
Iced Tea, Crystal Light Sugar Free, Raspberry	Kraft	8 fl. oz.	4
Ice Teasers, Citrus	Nestle	8 fl. oz.	6
Ice Teasers, Lemon	Nestle	8 fl. oz.	6
Ice Teasers, Orange	Nestle	8 fl. oz.	6
Ice Teasers, Tropical	Nestle	8 fl. oz.	6
Ice Teasers, Wild Cherry	Nestle	8 fl. oz.	6
Iced Berry Tea	Crystal Light	8 fl. oz.	3
Iced Tea	Shasta	12 fl. oz.	124
Iced Tea	Sipp's	8.45 fl. oz.	100

Withdraw from fatty foods slowly to ease the pain of separation.

Beverages

Product	Manufacturer	Serving Size	Calories
Iced Tea Mix	Nestle	8 fl. oz.	4
Iced Tea, Natural Lemon Flavor	Coca-Cola	8 fl. oz.	8
Instant Breakfast	Pillsbury	1 pouch	130
Instant Breakfast, Orange Pouch	Staff	6 fl. oz.	90
Instant Breakfast, Vanilla	Carnation	1 envelope	100
Instant Chocolate Milk Mix	Staff	2 tsp.	90
Instant Citrus Cooler	Gatorade	8 fl. oz.	60
Instant Fruit Punch	Gatorade	8 fl. oz.	60
Instant Lemon	Gatorade	8 fl. oz.	60
Kool-Aid, Black Cherry	Kraft	8 fl. oz.	2
Kool-Aid, Cherry	Kraft	8 fl. oz.	2
Kool-Aid, sugar free	Kraft	8 fl. oz.	3
Kool-Aid, Grape	Kraft	8 fl. oz.	3
Kool-Aid, Tropical Punch	Kraft	8 fl. oz.	2
Lager, Bohemian	Stroh's	12 fl. oz.	148
Lager, Signature	Stroh's	12 fl. oz.	150
Lemon Lime Cooler	Sipp's	8.45 fl. oz.	130
Lemon Lime Drink	Gatorade	8 fl. oz.	50
Lemonade	Sipp's	8.45 fl. oz.	85
Lemonade	generic	6 fl. oz.	80
Light Ale	Becks	12 fl. oz.	132
Light Berry Wine Cooler	Bartles & Jaymes	6 fl. oz.	75
Light Wine Cooler	Bartles & Jaymes	6 fl. oz.	67

Treat yourself well – you are important
and you are special.

Beverages

Product	Manufacturer	Serving Size	Calories
Limeaid	generic	6 fl. oz.	75
Limeaid, concentrate	generic	6 fl. oz.	410
Liqueur	Drambuie	1.5 fl. oz.	165
Liqueur	Pernod	1.5 fl. oz.	117
Liqueur	Southern Comfort	1.5 fl. oz.	180
Liqueur	Tia Maria	1.5 fl. oz.	138
Liqueur, anisette	generic	.75 fl. oz.	74
Liqueur, benedictine	generic	.75 fl. oz.	69
Liqueur, brandy-coffee	generic	1.5 fl. oz.	129
Liqueur, brandy–fruit flavored	generic	1.5 fl. oz.	129
Liqueur, cherry	generic	1.5 fl. oz.	120
Liqueur, coffee	generic	1.5 fl. oz.	174
Liqueur, creme de almonde	generic	1.5 fl. oz.	151
Liqueur, creme de banana	generic	1.5 fl. oz.	144
Liqueur, creme de cacao	generic	1.5 fl. oz.	150
Liqueur, creme de cassis	generic	1.5 fl. oz.	122
Liqueur, creme de menthe	generic	1.5 fl. oz.	186
Liqueur, distilled 100% proof	generic	1 fl. oz.	83
Liqueur, distilled 80% proof	generic	1 fl. oz.	67
Liqueur, distilled 84% proof	generic	1 fl. oz.	70

Food is the fuel your body needs to run on.

Beverages

Product	Manufacturer	Serving Size	Calories
Liqueur, distilled 86% proof	generic	1 fl. oz.	72
Liqueur, distilled 90% proof	generic	1 fl. oz.	75
Liqueur, distilled 94% proof	generic	1 fl. oz.	78
Liqueur, distilled 97% proof	generic	1 fl. oz.	81
Liqueur, peppermint schnapps	generic	1.5 fl. oz.	124
Madeira	generic	4 fl. oz.	160
Malt Liquor	Coqui	12 fl. oz.	200
Malt Liquor	Elephant	12 fl. oz.	211
Mineral water, unsweetened	generic	8 fl. oz.	0
Mix, Lemon Sour	Schweppe's	6 fl. oz.	75
Mix, Whiskey Sour	Schweppe's	2 fl. oz.	55
Mixed Berry Drink	Sipp's	8.45 fl. oz.	130
New Cranberry Breeze Low Calorie	Crystal Light	1/8 tub	5
O'Doul's, Non-Alcoholic Brew	Anheuser-Busch	12 fl. oz.	70
Orange Drink	Gatorade	8 fl. oz.	50
Orange Drink	Coca-Cola	8 fl. oz.	70
Ovaltine Classic	Sandoz	.75 oz.	80
Passion Fruit Drink	Welch's Orchard	6 fl. oz.	100
Picante Mild Flavor Canned Juice	Campbell's	6 fl. oz.	35
Pineapple Grapefruit	Ocean Spray	6 fl. oz.	110
Power Ade	Coca-Cola	8 fl. oz.	70

Your body can tell you which diet
is right for you – listen to it.

Beverages

Product	Manufacturer	Serving Size	Calories
Raspberry Cranberry Juice	Seneca	6 fl. oz.	110
Sharp's, Non-Alcoholic Brew	Miller	12 fl. oz.	58
Sherry	generic	2 fl. oz.	65
Soy Moo Soy Milk	Health Valley	1 cup	110
Sparkling Water	Seltzer	12 fl. oz.	0
Sparkling Water, Lemon-Lime Flavor	Canada Dry	6 fl. oz.	0
Sparkling Water, Raspberry Flavor	Canada Dry	6 fl. oz.	0
Spirit	Bacardi	2.5 fl. oz.	118
Splash, Fruit Sparkler	Ocean Spray	6 fl. oz.	100
Splash, Ruby Red Grapefruit	Ocean Spray	6 fl. oz.	100
Strawberry Drink	Ocean Spray	6 fl. oz.	110
Sunshine Punch Drink	Sipp's	8.45 fl. oz.	130
Tea, 100% Instant, as prepared	Nestle	8 fl. oz.	2
Tea, Crystal Light, sugar free	Kraft	8 fl. oz.	4
Tea, Crystal Light, sugar free, Grapefruit	Kraft	8 fl. oz.	4
Tea, decaffeinated	Lipton	8 fl. oz.	4
Tea, decaffeinated w/Nutrasweet	Lipton	8 fl. oz.	5
Tea, herbal bags, all flavors	Lipton	1 bag	4
Tea, Instant	Maxwell House	6 fl. oz.	2
Tea, lemon flavor	Nestle	8 fl. oz.	70
Tea, sugar free	Lipton	8 fl. oz.	1

Fructose is an ultra-refined sugar.

Beverages

Product	Manufacturer	Serving Size	Calories
Tonic Water	Schweppe's	8 fl. oz.	90
Tonic Water, diet	Canada Dry	6 fl. oz.	2
Tonic Water, low calorie	Schweppe's	8 fl. oz.	0
Tropical Fruit Drink	Gatorade	8 fl. oz.	50
Tropical Fruits Drink	Hawaiian Punch	6 fl. oz.	90
Tropical Squeeze Drink	Chiquita	6 fl. oz.	90
Verry Berry Drink	Hawaiian Punch	6 fl. oz.	90
Vichy Water	Schweppe's	6 fl. oz.	0
Water, Natural Spring	Evian	8 fl. oz.	0
Wild Fruit Drink	Hawaiian Punch	6 fl. oz.	90
Wine, Chablis	generic	4 fl. oz.	84
Wine, Chardonnay	generic	4 fl. oz.	88
Wine, Chenin Blanc	generic	4 fl. oz.	86
Wine, Chianti	generic	4 fl. oz.	100
Wine, Diet Chablis, California Cellars	Taylor	100 ml.	38
Wine, Light Blush	AlmandenVineyards	100 ml.	60
Wine, Light Chablis	AlmandenVineyards	100 ml.	55
Wine, Light Strawberry Splash	Seagrams	12 fl. oz.	120
Wine, Light, California Cellars	Taylor	100 ml.	54
Wine, Light, California Cellars, Blush	Taylor	100 ml.	58
Wine, Light Chablis	Taylor	100 ml.	55
Wine, Reisling	generic	4 fl. oz.	90
Wine, Rhine	generic	4 fl. oz.	96
Wine, Rhone	generic	4 fl. oz.	96

Common table salt is 40% sodium and 60% chloride.

Beverages

Product	Manufacturer	Serving Size	Calories
Wine, rose	generic	4 fl. oz.	90
Wine, Sauvignon Blanc	generic	4 fl. oz.	80
Wine, sherry dry	generic	4 fl. oz.	162
Wine, sweet	generic	4 fl. oz.	165
Wine, table red	generic	3.5 fl. oz.	74
Wine, table rose	generic	3.5 fl. oz.	73
Wine, table white	generic	3.5 fl. oz.	70
Wine, vermouth dry	generic	4 fl. oz.	136
Wine, vermouth sweet	generic	4 fl. oz.	180
Wine, white	Liebraumilch	4 fl. oz.	84

Poultry skin is high in fat.
Remove it before eating.

Bread

Product	Manufacturer	Serving Size	Calories
Bakery Light Country Bran Bread	Arnold's	1 slice	40
Bakery Light Golden Wheat Bread	Arnold's	1 slice	40
Bakery Light Italian Bread	Arnold's	1 slice	40
Bakery Light Oatmeal Bread	Arnold's	1 slice	40
Bakery Light Soft Rye Bread	Arnold's	1 slice	40
Light Sourdough Bread	Arnold's	1 slice	40
Light Style, FF, 7 Grain Bread	Pepperidge Farm	1 slice	40
Light Style, FF, Oatmeal Bread	Pepperidge Farm	1 slice	40
Light Style, FF, Vienna Bread	Pepperidge Farms	1 slice	40
Light Style, FF, Wheat Bread	Pepperidge Farms	1 slice	40
Nature's Own, Light Sourdough	Flowers	1 slice	40
Wheat, Thin Sliced	Pepperidge Farms	1 slice	35
White, Very Thin Sliced	Pepperidge Farms	1 slice	40
Cinnamon Roll	Sara Lee	1 roll	230
Croissant	Sara Lee	1 croissant	170
Danish – Apple	Sara Lee	1 danish	120
FF, Apple Cinnamon	Toast & Jammer's	1 piece	165
FF, Apple Cinnamon Twist	Entenmann's	1.1 oz.	90
FF, Apple Spice Cake	Entenmann's	1 oz.	70

Choose poached, steamed, or boiled fish instead
of breaded, battered, and fried.

Breakfast Breads

Product	Manufacturer	Serving Size	Calories
FF, Apricot Twist	Entenmann's	1.1 oz.	90
FF, Blueberry	Toast & Jammer's	1 piece	165
FF, Blueberry-Crunch Cake	Entenmann's	1 oz.	70
FF, Breakfast Bar, Apple	Health Valley	1 bar	110
FF, Breakfast Bar, Apricot	Health Valley	1 bar	110
FF, Breakfast Bar, Blueberry	Health Valley	1 bar	100
FF, Breakfast Bar, Cherry	Health Valley	1 bar	110
FF, Breakfast Bar, Raspberry	Health Valley	1 bar	110
FF, Breakfast Bar, Strawberry	Health Valley	1 bar	110
FF, Cheese Filled Crumb Coffee Cake	Entenmann's	1.3 oz.	90
FF, Cherry Cheese Coffee Cake	Entenmann's	1.3 oz.	90
FF, Cinnamon Twist	Entenmann's	1 oz.	80
FF, Fruit Muffin, Apple Spice	Health Valley	1 each	130
FF, Fruit Muffin, Banana	Health Valley	1 each	130
FF, Fruit Muffin, Raisin Spice	Health Valley	1 each	140
FF, Golden French Crumb Cake	Entenmann's	1 oz.	80
FF, Lemon Twist	Entenmann's	1.1 oz.	80

Control your food. Do not be controlled by food.

Breakfast Breads

Product	Manufacturer	Serving Size	Calories
FF, Louisiana Crunch Cake	Entenmann's	1 oz.	80
FF, Raspberry	Toast & Jammer's	1 piece	165
FF, Raspberry Twist	Entenmann's	1.1 oz.	90
FF, Strawberry	Toast & Jammer's	1 piece	165
Toastettes, Frosted Blueberry	Nabisco	1 piece	190

Food and drink are fuels – not your friends,
not your enemies.

Candies and Desserts

Product	Manufacturer	Serving Size	Calories
All FlavorsIce	Bresler's	3.5 oz.	120
Angel Food Chocolate Cake	General Mills	1/2 cake	150
Angel Food Confetti Cake	General Mills	1/2 cake	160
Angel Food Lemon Custard Cake	General Mills	1/2 cake	150
Angel Food Strawberry Cake	General Mills	1/2 cake	150
Angel Food Traditional Cake	General Mills	1/2 cake	130
Angel Food White Cake	General Mills	1/2 cake	150
Banana Creme Pudding	Royal	1/2 cup	80
Blow Pop, Assorted	Charm's Company	1 pop	50
Bonjour Non-Fat Frozen Yogurt	Colombo	4 oz.	100
Breath Savers	Breath Savers	1 candy	2
Breath Savers, Cinnamon	Breath Savers	1 candy	2
Breath Savers, Spearmint	Breath Savers	1 candy	2
Breath Savers, Wintergreen	Breath Savers	1 candy	2
Bubble Gum, Big Red	Life Savers	1 stick	10
Bubble Gum, diet, sugar-free	Extra	1 piece	7
Bubble-Yum, regular	Life Savers	1 piece	25
Bubble-Yum, sugar-free	Life Savers	1 piece	20

Think smart. Think healthy.

Candies and Desserts

Product	Manufacturer	Serving Size	Calories
Butterscotch Disks	Brach's	1 oz.	110
Butterscotch Pudding	Royal	1/2 cup	90
Candy Canes, Cinnamon	Bob's Candies, Inc.	1 piece	80
Candy Corn	Brach's	1 oz.	100
Candy Corn	generic	1 oz.	105
Candy Jar Peppermint Sweetwists	Bob's Candies, Inc.	2 pieces	50
Candy, hard	generic	1 oz.	110
Cherry & Apple Holiday Candy	Jolly Rancher	3 pieces	60
Cherry Orange Ice Stripes	Good Humor	1.5 oz.	35
Chocolate Pudding	Royal	1/2 cup	90
Chocolate Treat Bar, sugar free	Weight Watchers	1 oz.	90
Christmas Lollipops	Life Savers	1 candy	40
Cinnamon Disks	Brock Candy Co.	1 oz.	110
Cinnamon Disks	Brach's	1 oz.	110
Cinnamon Imperials	Brach's	1 oz.	110
Circus Peanuts	Brach's	1 oz.	100
Circus Peanuts	Brock Candy Co.	1 oz.	100
Creme Glace Chocolate	Avari	1 oz.	10
Creme Glace Chocolate	Gise	4 oz.	34
Creme Glace, All Flavors	Avari	1 oz.	10
Creme Glace, All Flavors	Gise	4 oz.	33
Custard Dessert Mix	Royal	1/2 cup	60
Dark-N-Sweet Chocolate	Royal	1/2 cup	90
Desert Spice	Nile Spice	1/8 tsp.	0

Take that weight off your mind.

Candies and Desserts

Product	Manufacturer	Serving Size	Calories
Dessert Bar, Choc. Fudge Swirl	Sealtest Free	1 bar	90
Dessert Mints	Brach's	1 oz.	110
Dessert, Choc. Frozen Swirl, FF	Weight Watchers	1/2 cup	90
Dutch Chocolate	American Glace	4 oz.	48
Dutch Chocolate Bar	American Glace	4 oz.	48
Easter Pops	Life Savers	1 candy	40
FF, Black Cherry Frozen Dessert	Sealtest Free	1/2 cup	100
FF, Chocolate Frozen Yogurt	Sealtest Free	1/2 cup	100
FF, Chocolate Vanilla Twist	Baskin Robbin's	1/2 cup	100
FF, Chocolate Frozen Dessert	Weight Watchers	1/2 cup	80
FF, Frozen Dessert, Chocolate	Sealtest Free	1/2 cup	100
FF, Just Peachy	Baskin Robbin's	1/2 cup	100
FF, Marble Fudge Frozen Dessert	Edy's	4 oz.	100
FF, Natural Black Cherry, Frozen Dessert	Sealtest Free	1/2 cup	100
FF, Natural Red Raspberry, Frozen Dessert	Sealtest Free	1/2 cup	100
FF, Natural Strawberry, Frozen Dessert	Sealtest Free	1/2 cup	100
FF, Snack Pack Pudding, Vanilla	Hunt's	4 oz.	100
FF, Strawberry, Frozen Dessert	Sealtest Free	1/2 cup	90

Buy meat with as little marbling as possible.

Candies and Desserts

Product	Manufacturer	Serving Size	Calories
FF, Vanilla Frozen Dessert	Edy's	4 oz.	90
FF, Vanilla Frozen Yogurt	Sealtest Free	1/2 cup	100
Fancy Fruit	Life Savers	1 candy	8
Flan Caramel Custard	Royal	1/2 cup	60
Fluffy White Frosting Mix	Pillsbury	1/2 cake	60
Fondant, uncooked	generic	1 oz.	105
Frost It Hot Chocolate	Pillsbury	1/2 cake	50
Frost It Hot Fluffy White	Pillsbury	1/2 cake	50
Frozen Delight Fudge Bar	Ultra Slim Fast	1 bar	70
Fruit & Juice Bar, Cherry	Chiquita	1 bar	50
Fruit & Juice Bar, Raspberry	Chiquita	1 bar	50
Fruit & Juice Bar, Raspberry/Banana	Chiquita	1 bar	50
Fruit & Juice Bar, Strawberry	Chiquita	1 bar	50
Fruit & Juice Bar, Strawberry/Banana	Chiquita	1 bar	50
Fruit & Juice Bar	Welch's	1 bar	25
Fruit Bunch	Brach's	1 oz.	90
Fruit Juicers, Citrus Fruits	Life Savers	1 candy	8
Fruit Juicers, Easter Egg Assortment	Life Savers	1 candy	10
Fruit Juicers, Fruit Punch	Life Savers	1 candy	8
Fruit Juicers, Grape	Life Savers	1 candy	8

Avoid high-fat processed meat products, such as
salami, bacon, bologna, and frankfurters.

Candies and Desserts

Product	Manufacturer	Serving Size	Calories
Fruit Juicers, Lollipops	Life Savers	1 candy	40
Fruit Juicers, Strawberry	Life Savers	1 candy	8
Funmallows	Kraft	1	30
Gelatin Dessert, Apple	Royal	1/2 cup	80
Gelatin Dessert, Apricot	Jell-0	1/2 cup	80
Gelatin Dessert, Black Cherry	Jell-O	1/2 cup	80
Gelatin Dessert, Blackberry	Royal	1/2 cup	80
Gelatin Dessert, Blueberry	Jell-O	1/2 cup	80
Gelatin Dessert, Cherry	Jell-O	1/2 cup	80
Gelatin Dessert, Concord Grape	Royal	1/2 cup	80
Gelatin Dessert, Grape	Jell-O	1/2 cup	80
Gelatin Dessert, Lemon	Jell-O	1/2 cup	80
Gelatin Dessert, Lemon	Royal	1/2 cup	80
Gelatin Dessert, Lemon-Lime	Royal	1/2 cup	80
Gelatin Dessert, Lime	Jell-O	1/2 cup	80
Gelatin Dessert, Lime	Royal	1/2 cup	80
Gelatin Dessert, Mixberry	Royal	1/2 cup	80
Gelatin Dessert, Mixed Fruit	Jell-O	1/2 cup	80
Gelatin Dessert, Orange	Jell-O	1/2 cup	80
Gelatin Dessert, Orange	Royal	1/2 cup	80
Gelatin Dessert, Peach	Jell-O	1/2 cup	80
Gelatin Dessert, Peach	Royal	1/2 cup	80

Liver is a good source of iron.

Candies and Desserts

Product	Manufacturer	Serving Size	Calories
Gelatin Dessert, Pineapple	Royal	1/2 cup	80
Gelatin Dessert, as prepared	generic	1/2 cup	70
Gelatin Dessert, Raspberry	Royal	1/2 cup	80
Gelatin Dessert, Strawberry	Jell-O	1/2 cup	80
Gelatin Dessert, Strawberry	Royal	1/2 cup	80
Gelatin Dessert, Strawberry/Banana	Jell-O	1/2 cup	80
Gelatin Dessert, sugar-free Cherry	Royal	1/2 cup	8
Gelatin Dessert, sugar-free Lime	Royal	1/2 cup	8
Gelatin Dessert, sugar-free Orange	Royal	1/2 cup	10
Gelatin Dessert, sugar-free Raspberry	Royal	1/2 cup	8
Gelatin Dessert, sugar-free Strawberry	Royal	1/2 cup	8
Gelatin Dessert, Tropical Punch	Jell-O	1/2 cup	80
Gelatin Dessert, Watermelon	Jell-O	1/2 cup	80
Gelatin Dessert, Wild Strawberry	Jell-O	1/2 cup	80
Gelatin, dry	generic	1 envelope	25
Gelatin, Fruit Flavored	Royal	1/2 cup	70
Gelatin, Lite, Black Cherry	Four Winds	1/2 cup	100

Broil or bake, instead of frying.

Candies and Desserts

Product	Manufacturer	Serving Size	Calories
Gelatin, Lite, Blueberry	Four Winds	1/2 cup	100
Gelatin, Lite, Peach	Four Winds	1/2 cup	100
Gelatin, Lite, Raspberry	Four Winds	1/2 cup	100
Gelatin, Lite, Strawberry	Four Winds	1/2 cup	100
Gelatin, Lite, Strawberry/Banana	Four Winds	3.5 oz.	80
Gelatin, Raspberry/Strawberry/Banana	Jell-O	3.5 oz.	80
Gelatin, Strawberry sugar-free	Royal	1/2 cup	8
Gelatin, Strawberry/Banana, sugar-free	Jell-O	4 oz.	8
Gelatin, Strawberry/Orange	Jell-O	3.5 oz.	80
Gelatin, Strawberry/Orange	Royal	1/2 cup	80
Gelatin, Tropical Fruit	Royal	1/2 cup	80
Giant Mint Stick	American Candy Co.	1/9 stick	80
Glitters	Brock Candy Co.	1 oz.	110
Grape Lemon Ice Stripes	Good Humor	1.5 oz.	35
Gum	Juicy Fruit	1 stick	10
Gum Drops	generic	1 oz.	100
Gum, Blueberry	Hubba-Bubba	1 piece	23
Gum, candy-coated pieces	generic	12 pieces	63
Gum, chewing, Bubble Gum	Carefree	1 piece	10

Don't be a victim, be a survivor.

Candies and Desserts

Product	Manufacturer	Serving Size	Calories
Gum, chewing, Bubble Gum	Fruit Stripe	1 piece	8
Gum, chewing, Cinnamon	Beech Nut	1 piece	10
Gum, chewing, Fruit	Beech Nut	1 piece	10
Gum, chewing, Fruit-n-Juicy	Bubble Yum	1 piece	20
Gum, chewing, Luscious Lime	Bubble Yum	1 piece	25
Gum, chewing, Peppermint	Beech Nut	1 piece	10
Gum, chewing, sugarless	Carefree	1 piece	8
Gum, chewing, Variety pack	Fruit Stripe	1 piece	8
Gum, Cinnamon	Freedent	1 stick	10
Gum, Cola	Hubba-Bubba	1 piece	23
Gum, Diet, Cinnamon, sugar free	Extra	1 piece	8
Gum, Diet, Peppermint, sugar free	Extra	1 piece	10
Gum, Diet Spearmint, sugar free	Extra	1 piece	8
Gum, Diet, Winter Fresh, sugar free	Extra	1 piece	8
Gum, Doublemint	Wrigley's	1 stick	10
Gum, Fruit Stripe, all flavors	Freedent	1 stick	10
Gum, Grape	Hubba-Bubba	1 piece	23
Gum, Grape, sugar free	Hubba-Bubba	1 piece	13

Examine your eating habits.

Candies and Desserts

Product	Manufacturer	Serving Size	Calories
Gum, Original	Hubba-Bubba	1 piece	23
Gum, Original, sugar free	Hubba-Bubba	1 piece	14
Gum, Peppermint	Freedent	1 stick	10
Gum, Raspberry	Freedent	1 piece	23
Gum, Spearmint	Freedent	1 stick	10
Gum, Spearmint	Wrigley's	1 stick	10
Gum, Strawberry	Hubba-Bubba	1 piece	23
Gumi Bears	Brach's	1 oz.	100
Gummi Savers, Grape	Life Savers	1 candy	12
Gummi Savers, Mixed Berry	Life Savers	1 candy	12
Gummi Worms	Brach's	1 oz.	100
Gummy Bears	Estee	3 pieces	20
Gummy Squirms, Old World Gummy Snacks	Brock Candy Co.	1 oz.	100
Hard Candy	Estee	2 pieces	25
Holes, Sunshine Fruits	Life Savers	1 candy	2
Holes, Tangerine	Life Savers	1 candy	2
Holiday Marshmallow, Vanilla	Kraft	1/2 cup	100
Hot Fudge, FF, sugar free	Johnston's	1.5 oz.	84
Ice Cream Topping, Caramel	Kraft	1 Tbsp.	60
Ice Cream Topping, Chocolate	Kraft	1 Tbsp.	50
Ice Cream Topping, Chocolate Syrup	Smucker's	2 Tbsp.	130

Fat is the most concentrated calorie source.

Candies and Desserts

Product	Manufacturer	Serving Size	Calories
Ice Cream Topping, Hot Fudge	Kraft	1 Tbsp.	70
Ice Cream Topping, Marshmallow Creme	Kraft	1 Tbsp.	90
Ice Cream Topping, Marshmallow	Smucker's	2 Tbsp.	120
Ice Cream Topping, Pineapple	Kraft	1 Tbsp.	50
Ice Cream Topping, Pineapple	Smucker's	2 Tbsp.	130
Ice Cream Topping, Strawberry	Kraft	1 Tbsp.	50
Ice Cream Topping, Strawberry	Smucker's	2 Tbsp.	120
Inspirations, Non-Fat Frozen Yogurt, Chocolate	Edy's	4 oz.	90
Inspirations, Non-Fat Frozen Yogurt, Raspberry	Edy's	4 oz.	90
Inspirations, Non-Fat Frozen Yogurt, Strawberry	Edy's	4 oz.	90
Inspirations, Non-Fat Frozen Yogurt, Vanilla	Edy's	4 oz.	100
Jellie Beans	Brach's	1 oz.	100
Jellie Beans	generic	1 oz.	105
Jelly Beans	Brock Candy Co.	12 pieces	140
Jelly Belly	generic	2.5 oz.	140
Jelly Belly 39, Assorted Flavors	Herman Goelitz Candy Co.	2 oz.	220
Jube Jels	Brach's	1 oz.	100
Just 10, Frozen Dessert sugar free, non-fat	Honey Hill Farms	1 oz.	10

Reducing fat intake is one of the
most effective ways to cut calories.

Candies and Desserts

Product	Manufacturer	Serving Size	Calories
Kentucky Mints	Brach's	1 oz.	100
Key Lime Pie Filling	Royal	1/2 cup	50
Lemon Drops	Brach's	1 oz.	100
Lemon Drops	Brock Candy Co.	1 oz.	110
Lemon Ice Frozen Dessert	Ben & Jerry's	4 oz.	105
Lemon-Pie Filling	Royal	1/2 cup	50
Life Savers Ice Pops	Life Savers	1 ice pop	35
Life Savers Ice Pops, sugar free	Life Savers	1 ice pop	12
Lollipops	Estee	1 piece	25
Lollipops, all flavors	Life Savers	1 piece	45
Lollydrops	Brach's	1 oz.	100
Marshmallow Miniatures	Kraft	10	18
Marshmallows, Campfire	Borden	2 pieces	40
Marshmallows, Holiday Vanilla	Kraft	1/2 cup	100
Marshmallows, Jet Puffed	Kraft	1 piece	25
Mint Coolers	Brach's	1 oz.	100
Neopolitan, FF, Frozen Dessert	Weight Watchers	1/2 cup	80
Non-Fat Frozen Yogurt, Fudge Marble	Kemps	3 fl. oz.	80
Non-Fat Frozen Yogurt, Natural Peach	Sealtest	1/2 cup	100
Non-Fat Frozen Yogurt, Strawberry	Kemps	3 fl. oz.	70
Non-Fat Frozen Yogurt, Strawberry	Sealtest	1/2 cup	100

A low fat and cholesterol diet is the first
step to lowering blood cholesterol.

Candies and Desserts

Product	Manufacturer	Serving Size	Calories
Non-Fat Frozen Yogurt, Vanilla	Kemps	3 fl. oz.	70
Olde Timey Peppermint Candy	Bob's Candies Inc.	1/2 oz.	16
Orange Slices	Brock Candy Co.	5 pieces	140
Orange-Vanilla Treat Bar, FF, sugar free	Weight Watchers	1 bar	30
Orangettes	Brach's	1 oz.	100
Party Mints	Kraft	1 mint	8
Passion Fruit Dessert	Vitari	4 oz.	80
Peach Dessert	Vitari	4 oz.	80
Peach, Frozen Dessert	Sealtest Free	1/2 cup	100
Peppermint Starlight Mints	Brach's	1 oz.	100
Perky's Gummi Bears	Brach's	1 oz.	100
Pixy Stick	Sunmark Inc. Co.	1 straw	8
Pound Cake, Free & Light	Sara Lee	1 slice	70
Pudding, FF, Chocolate/Vanilla	Hershey's	4 oz.	100
Pudding, Vanilla	Royal	2 Tbsp.	50
Pudding, French Vanilla & Lemon	Jell-O	1/2 cup	90
Raspberry Sorbet, Frozen Dessert	Fausen Gladie	1/2 cup	140
Red Twists	Brach's	1 oz.	100
Royal Lites, Frozen Desserts all flavors	Bresler's	4 oz.	217
Sea Tarts, tangy candy	Sunmark Inc. Co.	1 roll	25

A small amount of fat is necessary for certain body functions and to help absorb certain vitamins.

Candies and Desserts

Product	Manufacturer	Serving Size	Calories
Skinny Dip Ice Cream	Skinny Dip	4 oz.	36
Smarties	Brock Candy Co.	1 oz.	100
Snappytarts	Brach's	1 oz.	100
Sorbet, mandarin orange	generic	4 oz.	110
Sorbet, peach	generic	4 oz.	120
Sorbet, pineapple	generic	4 oz.	120
Sorbet, raspberry	generic	4 oz.	110
Sour Balls	Brach's	1 oz.	100
Sour Balls	Brock Candy Co.	1 oz.	110
Sour Gummi Cave Creatures	Brach's	1 oz.	100
Sour Gummi Sea Creatures	Brach's	1 oz.	100
Sparkles Starlight Mints	Brach's	1 oz.	100
Spearmint Leaves	Brach's	1 oz.	100
Spearmint Starlight Mints	Brach's	1 oz.	110
Spice Drops	Brock Candy Co.	12 pieces	130
Spicettes	Brach's	1 oz.	100
Starlight Mints	Brock Candy Co.	3 pieces	60
Strawberry Ice Frozen Dessert	Ben & Jerry's	4 oz.	77
Sugar-Free Candy	Life Savers	1 piece	8
Sunshine Fruits	Life Savers	1 candy	8
Tahitian Vanilla	American Glace	4 oz.	48
Tropical Fruits	Life Savers	1 candy	8
Valentine Pops	Life Savers	1 candy	40
Vanilla Fudge Royal	Sealtest Free	1/2 cup	100
Vanilla Sandwich Dessert Bar, FF	Weight Watchers	1 bar	130

Diet + Exercise = Health

Candies and Desserts

Product	Manufacturer	Serving Size	Calories
Vanilla Strawberry Royal	Sealtest Free	1/2 cup	100
Vanilla, FF, Fzn. Dessert	Weight Watchers	1/2 cup	80
Vanilla-Fudge Swirl Dessert Bar	Sealtest Free	1 bar	80
Velamints	Kraft	1 mint	8
Velamints, Cocomints	Kraft	1 mint	8
Wild Cherry	Life Savers	1 candy	8
Yogurt, Blended, Blueberry/Strawberry	Dannon	4.4 oz.	120
Yogurt, Blended, French Vanilla	Dannon	3/4 cup	150
Yogurt, Blended	Dannon	4.4 oz.	110
Yogurt, Cherries Jubilee, Ultimate 90	Weight Watchers	1 cup	90
Yogurt, FF, Black Cherry 70	Light N' Lively	6 oz.	70
Yogurt, FF, Blueberry 70	Light N' Lively	6 oz.	70
Yogurt, FF, Cherry	Yoplait	6 oz.	170
Yogurt, FF, Lemon 70	Light N' Lively	6 oz.	70
Yogurt, FF, Light, Blueberry/Strawberry	Dannon	4.4 oz.	50
Yogurt, FF, Light Cherry	Yoplait	6 oz.	90
Yogurt, FF, Peach	Yoplait	6 oz.	170
Yogurt, FF, Peach 70	Light N' Lively	6 oz.	70
Yogurt, FF, Peach/Strawberry	Dannon	4.4 oz.	50
Yogurt, FF, Strawberry	Yoplait	6 oz.	170

A healthy body = A healthy mind.

Candies and Desserts

Product	Manufacturer	Serving Size	Calories
Yogurt, FF, Strawberry 70	Light N' Lively	6 oz.	70
Yogurt, FF, Strawberry Fruitcup	Light N' Lively	6 oz.	70
Yogurt, FF, Strawberry-Banana	Light N' Lively	6 oz.	70
Yogurt, FF, Strawberry-Banana	Yoplait	6 oz.	170
Yogurt, Light, Cherry-Vanilla Single Serving	Dannon	8 oz.	100
Yogurt, Light, Lemon-Chiffon Single Serving	Dannon	8 oz.	100
Yogurt, Light, Peach Single Serving	Dannon	8 oz.	100
Yogurt, Light, Raspberry Single Serving	Dannon	8 oz.	100
Yogurt, Light, Straw-Fruit Cup Single Serving	Dannon	8 oz.	100
Yogurt, Light, Strawberry Single Serving	Dannon	8 oz.	100
Yogurt, Peach, Ultimate 90	Weight Watchers	1 cup	90
Yogurt, Raspberry, Frozen, non-fat	Carnation	4 oz.	110
Yogurt, Strawberry, Frozen, non-fat	Baskin Robbin's	1/2 cup	110
Yogurt, Strawberry, Frozen, non-fat	Carnation	4 oz.	110
Yogurt, Strawberry-Banana, Ultimate 90	Weight Watchers	1 cup	90
Zip-A-Dee-Doo-Da Pops	Charm's Company	3 pops	60

Choose a diet with plenty of vegetables, fruits, and grain products.

Cereals

Product	Manufacturer	Serving Size	Calories
All Bran Extra Fiber	Kellogg's	1/2 cup	50
Almond Flavor O's	Health Valley	1 oz.	100
Apple Cinnamon O's	Health Valley	1 oz.	100
Apple Cinnamon Squares	Kellogg's	1 oz.	90
Apple Jacks	Kellogg's	1 oz.	110
Apple Raisin Crisp	Kellogg's	1 oz.	130
Blueberry Squares	Kellogg's	1/2 cup	90
Bran Flakes	Kellogg's	1 oz.	90
Bran Flakes	Post	1 oz.	90
Cocoa Krispies	Kellogg's	3/4 cup	110
Corn Chex	Ralston	1 oz.	110
Cream of Rice	Nabisco	1 oz.	100
Cream of Wheat	Nabisco	1 oz.	100
Cream of Wheat, Instant	Nabisco	1 packet	100
Cream of Wheat, Quick	Nabisco	1 oz.	100
Crispix	Kellogg's	1 oz.	110
Double Chex	Ralston	1 oz.	100
Double-Dip Crunch	Kellogg's	2/3 cup	110
FF, Fruit Lites, Brown Rice	Health Valley	1/2 oz.	50
FF, Fruit Lites, Golden Corn	Health Valley	1/2 oz.	50
FF, Granola Date and Almond Flavor	Health Valley	1 oz.	90
FF, Granola, Raisin Cinnamon	Health Valley	1 oz.	90
FF, Granola, Tropical Fruit	Health Valley	1 oz.	90

Eat breakfast foods with lots of fiber.

Cereals

Product	Manufacturer	Serving Size	Calories
FF, High Fiber O's	Health Valley	1 oz.	100
Frosted Bran	Kellogg's	1 oz.	110
Frosted Flakes	Kellogg's	1 oz.	110
Frosted Krispies	Kellogg's	1 oz.	110
Frosted Mini Wheats, Bite Size	Kellogg's	1/2 cup	100
Frosted Mini Wheats	Kellogg's	1 oz.	100
Frosted Rice Chex Juniors	Ralston	1 oz.	110
Frosted Wheat Squares	Nabisco	1 oz.	100
Fruit Wheat Strawberry	Nabisco	1 oz.	90
Fruitful Bran	Kellogg's	1.4 oz.	120
Fruity Marshmallow Krispies	Kellogg's	1.3 oz.	140
Grape-Nut Flakes	Post	1 oz.	110
Grits, Instant	Jim Dandy	.8 oz.	80
Grits, Original	Quaker	3 Tbsp.	100
Grits, Quick	Quaker	3 Tbsp.	100
Honeycomb	Post	1 oz.	110
Instant Grits, Country Bacon	Quaker	1 oz.	100
Instant Grits, Sausage	Quaker	1 oz.	90
Multi Bran Chex	Ralston	1 oz.	90
Nutri-Grain, Wheat	Kellogg's	1 oz.	90
Fruit Spread, Light Strawberry	Smucker's	1 tsp.	7
Grape Spread, reduced calorie	Weight Watchers	1 tsp.	8
Grated Parmesan Italian Topping	Weight Watchers	1 Tbsp.	15

Only use salt, sodium, and sugar in moderation.

Cereals

Product	Manufacturer	Serving Size	Calories
Hot Fudge, FF, Light Toppings	Smucker's	2 Tbsp.	70
Jam, All Flavors	Smucker's	1 tsp.	18
Jam, Apricot	Country Pure	2 tsp.	35
Jam, Apricot	Mary Ellen	2 tsp.	35
Jam, Apricot-Pineapple reduced calorie	S + W	1 tsp.	4
Jam, Apricot	Bama	3.5 oz.	250
Jam, Blackberry	Bama	3.5 oz.	250
Jam, Blackberry	Country Pure	2 tsp.	35
Product 19	Kellogg's	1 oz.	100
Puffed Corn	Arrowhead	1/2 oz.	50
Puffed Millet	Arrowhead	1/2 oz.	50
Puffed Rice	Arrowhead	1/2 oz.	50
Puffed Wheat	Arrowhead	1/2 oz.	50
Puffed Wheat	Post	1/2 oz.	50
Raisin Squares	Kellogg's	1 oz.	90
Rice Chex	Ralston	1 oz.	110
Rice Krispies	Kellogg's	1 oz.	110
Shredded Wheat	Nabisco	1 piece	80
Shredded Wheat, In Bran	Nabisco	1 oz.	90
Special K	Kellogg's	1 oz.	110
Strawberry Squares	Kellogg's	1 oz.	90
Super Golden Crisp	Post	1 oz.	100
Whole Grain Wheat Cereal	Ralston	1 oz.	100
Whole Grain, Shredded Wheat	Kellogg's	1 oz.	90

The most common type of diabetes
occurs in overweight adults.

Condiments

Product	Manufacturer	Serving Size	Calories
All Purpose	McCormick/Schilling (spice blends)	1 tsp.	3
All Purpose Seafood Seasoning	Golden Dipt	1/4 tsp.	2
Allspice	generic	1 tsp.	5
Almond Extract	McCormick/Schilling	1 tsp.	10
Almond Extract	generic	1 tsp.	0
Almond Pure Extract	Durkee	1 tsp.	13
Anise Extract	Durkee	1 tsp.	16
Anise-Pure Extract	McCormick/ Schilling	1 tsp.	23
Aspartame Sweetener	Staff	1 pk.	4
Baby Kosher Dill Pickles	Heinz	1 oz.	4
Bacon & Onion	Lawry's (Spice Blends)	1 tsp.	10
Baking Powder, low sodium	generic	1 tsp.	5
Baking Soda	generic	1/2 tsp.	0
Balsamic Vinegar	generic	1 Tbsp.	2
Banana Flavor	Durkee	1 tsp.	15
Banana-Imitation Extract	McCormick/ Schilling	1 tsp.	11
Bar-B-Q Shaker	Diamond Crystal	1/2 tsp.	4
Barbecue Sauce	Bull's Eye	2 Tbsp.	50
Barbecue Sauce	Chri's & Pitt's	1 Tbsp.	15
Barbecue Sauce	Featherweight	1 Tbsp.	14
Barbecue Sauce	Staff	1 Tbsp.	25
Basil	generic	1 tsp.	4
Bayleaf	generic	1 leaf	2
Black Bean Dip, Mild	Guiltless Gourmet	1 oz.	25

Food is the fuel your body needs to run on.

Condiments

Product	Manufacturer	Serving Size	Calories
Black Bean Dip, Spicy	Guiltless Gourmet	1 oz.	25
Black Walnut Extract, Cold	McCormick/Schilling	1 tsp.	12
Black Walnut Extract, Heated	McCormick/Schilling	1 tsp.	1
Black Walnut Flavor	Durkee	1 tsp.	4
Blackened Red Fish Seasoning	Golden Dipt	1/4 tsp.	2
Brandy Extract	generic	1 tsp.	0
Brandy Flavor	Durkee	1 tsp.	15
Brandy-Imitation Extract	McCormick/Schilling	1 tsp.	20
Bread & Butter Pickle Chunks	Vlasic	1 oz.	25
Breading Frying Mix	Golden Dipt	1 oz.	90
Breakfast Syrup	Brer Rabbit	2 Tbsp.	100
Broiled Fish Seasoning	Golden Dipt	1/4 tsp.	2
Brown Sugar	Sweet 'N Low	1 tsp.	4
Brownulated Sugar	Domino	1 tsp.	12
Butter Flavor	Durkee	1 tsp.	3
Butter Flavor	McCormick/Schilling	1 tsp.	1
Cactus Salsa	Cisco Kid's	1/2 oz.	0
Cajun seasoning	generic	1 Tbsp.	17
Cajun Style Shrimp and Crab Seasoning	Golden Dipt	1/4 tsp.	2
Catsup	Estee	1 Tbsp.	6
Catsup	Heinz	1 Tbsp.	16
Catsup	Smucker's	1 tsp.	8

Eat smart. Eat slow.

Condiments

Product	Manufacturer	Serving Size	Calories
Catsup	Weight Watchers	2 tsp.	8
Catsup	generic	1 Tbsp.	15
Catsup, Hot	Heinz	1 Tbsp.	14
Catsup, Lite	Heinz	1 Tbsp.	8
Cattleman's Mild Barbecue Sauce	French's	1 Tbsp.	25
Cattleman's Smokey Barbecue Sauce	French's	1 Tbsp.	25
Cayenne Pepper	generic	1 tsp.	6
Cheddar Queso, Spicy	Guiltless Gourmet	1 oz.	22
Chef Seasoning	Diamond Crystal	1 pkg.	2
Chef Shaker	Diamond Crystal	1/2 tsp.	4
Cherry Extract	Durkee	1 tsp.	3
Chicken granules	generic	1 tsp.	9
Chili sauce	generic	1 Tbsp.	16
Chili powder	generic	1 tsp.	10
Chipotle Salsa	Cisco Kid's	1/2 oz.	6
Chives, chopped	generic	1 tsp.	0.33
Chocolate Extract, cold	McCormick/ Schilling	1 tsp.	0
Chocolate Extract, heated	McCormick/ Schilling	1 tsp.	2
Chocolate Flavor	Durkee	1 tsp.	7
Cider vinegar	generic	1 tsp.	0
Cilantro, chopped	generic	1 Tbsp.	1
Cinnamon	generic	1 tsp.	5
Cinnamon stick	generic	1 stick	0
Cleopatra's Secret Seasoning	Nile Spice	1/8 tsp.	0

Exercise care in selecting your food. Maintain a balanced diet.

Condiments

Product	Manufacturer	Serving Size	Calories
Cloves, whole	generic	1 tsp.	0
Cocktail onions	generic	1/2 cup	21
Coconut flavor	Durkee	1 tsp.	8
Coconut-Imitation Extract	McCormick/Schilling	1 tsp.	7
Coriander	generic	1 tsp.	2
Corn starch	generic	1 Tbsp.	30
Corny Dog Batter	Golden Dipt	1 oz.	100
Creme De Menthe Extract	Durkee	1 tsp.	9
Crunchy Dill Pickles (no garlic)	Vlasic	1 oz.	4
Curry powder	generic	1 Tbsp.	15
Dark Molasses	Brer Rabbit	2 Tbsp.	110
Dark Syrup	Brer Rabbit	2 Tbsp.	110
Deli Bread & Butter Pickles (refrigerated)	Vlasic	1 oz.	25
Deli Pickle Halves (refrigerated)	Vlasic	1 oz.	4
Deli Style Dill Pickle Halves	Del Monte	1 oz.	4
Dijon Mustard	Grey Poupon	1 tsp.	6
Dill Pickle Halves	Del Monte	1 oz.	3
Dill pickle slices	generic	4 slices	0.6
Dill Pickle Spears (no garlic)	Vlasic	1 oz.	4
Dill Pickles	Claussen	1 oz.	6
Dill Pickles	Del Monte	1 medium	15
Dill weed	generic	1 tsp.	3
Dried chili peppers	generic	1 tsp.	0

Eat, drink, and be merry, for tomorrow we exercise.

Condiments

Product	Manufacturer	Serving Size	Calories
Dried grated lemon peel	generic	1 Tbsp.	0
Dried lemon peel	generic	1 tsp.	0
Dried parsley	generic	1 Tbsp.	12
Dry hot mustard	generic	1 tsp.	0
Dry mustard	generic	1 tsp.	0
Extra Spicy	Mrs. Dash (spice blends)	1 tsp.	12
FF, Black Bean Dip	Cisco Kid's	1/2 oz.	10
FF, Jalapeno Spread	Hain	1 oz.	30
FF, Tomato Salsa	Cisco Kid's	1/2 oz.	0
FF, Vegetable Broth, Cheese Spread	Hain	1 oz.	30
Fluid Sweetener	Sweet 'N Low	10 drops	0
French Shaker	Diamond Crystal	1/2 tsp.	4
Fresh basil	generic	1 tsp.	0
Fresh dill	generic	1 tsp.	0
Fresh mild salsa	generic	1 cup	70
Garlic clove	generic	1 clove	4.33
Garlic Pepper	Lawry's (Spice Blends)	1/4 tsp.	2
Garlic powder	generic	1 tsp.	10
Garlic powder	generic	1 Tbsp.	30
Garlic Powder, with parsley	Lawry's (Spice Blends)	1 tsp.	12
Garlic Salt	Lawry's (Spice Blends)	1 tsp.	4
Garlic, saltless	McCormick/Schilling (spice blends)	1 tsp.	11
Genuine Dill Pickles	generic	1 oz.	2

You are what you eat.

Condiments

Product	Manufacturer	Serving Size	Calories
Gherkin Pickles	generic	1 small	22
Ginger	generic	1 tsp.	6
Ginger Curry Seasoning	Nile Spice	1/8 tsp.	0
Ginger, fresh	generic	1 Tbsp.	9
Golden Light Brown Sugar	Domino	1 tsp.	16
Grated Lemon Peel	generic	1 Tbsp.	0
Grated Lime Peel	generic	1 Tbsp.	0
Grated Orange Rind	generic	1 Tbsp.	0
Green Chili Sauce, Hot	El Molino	2 Tbsp.	10
Green Food Coloring	generic	few drops	0
Ground Coriander	generic	1 tsp.	2
Hamburger Dill Pickle Chips (1/2 the salt)	Vlasic	1 oz.	2
Hamburger Dill Pickles	generic	1 oz.	2
Hamburger Pickle Chips	generic	1 oz.	2
Healthy Favorites, Hickory Smoke Barbecue Sauce	Kraft	2 Tbsp.	50
Healthy Favorites, Orig. Barbecue Sauce	Kraft	2 Tbsp.	50
Hickory Barbecue Sauce	Healthy Choice	2 Tbsp.	30
Hickory Barbecue Sauce	Staff	1 Tbsp.	30
Honey	generic	1 tsp.	22
Honey	Golden Blossom	1 Tbsp.	20
Honey	Smucker's	1 cup	1030
Honey	Smucker's	1 Tbsp.	65
Honey, Clover	Burleson	1 Tbsp.	60

Change your eating habits.
Try new, healthier products.

Condiments

Product	Manufacturer	Serving Size	Calories
Honey, Creamed	Burleson	1 Tbsp.	60
Honey, Natural	Burleson	1 Tbsp.	60
Honey, pure	Burleson	1 Tbsp.	60
Honey, raw	Burleson	1 Tbsp.	60
Honey, Rocky Mountain Clover	Burleson	1 Tbsp.	60
Honey, Single Serving	Smucker's	1/2 oz.	45
Honey, strained or extracted	generic	1 Tbsp.	65
Honey, strained or extracted	generic	1 cup	1030
Horseradish	generic	1 Tbsp.	6
Horseradish Root	generic	1 Tbsp.	2
Hot Garlic Pickles	generic	1 oz.	6
Hot Green Chili Salsa	Ortega	1 Tbsp.	6
Hot Green Chilis	generic	1 cup	40
Hot Picante Sauce	Guiltless Gourmet	1 oz.	6
Hot Salsa	Newman's Own	2 Tbsp.	10
Hot 'N Spicy Seasoned Salt	Lawry's (Spice Blends)	1 tsp.	3
Hush Puppy Deluxe Mix	Golden Dipt	1 1/4 oz.	120
Hush Puppy Deluxe Mix with Onion	Golden Dipt	1 1/4 oz.	120
Instant Dissolving Sugar	Domino	1 tsp.	16
It's a Dilly	McCormick/Schilling (spice blends)	1 tsp.	11
Italian Shaker	Diamond Crystal	1/2 tsp.	4

Juice your vegetables.
Learn new ways to approach food.

Condiments

Product	Manufacturer	Serving Size	Calories
Italian spices	generic	1 tsp.	5
Jalapeno Flavored Bean Sauce	Wise	2 Tbsp.	25
Jalapeno, Sliced	Trappey's	1 oz.	6
Jam, Jams & Preserves	generic	1 Tbsp.	55
Jellies	generic	1 Tbsp.	50
Kosher Baby Dill Pickles	Vlasic	1 oz.	4
Kosher Crunchy Dill Pickles (1/2 the salt)	Vlasic	1 oz.	4
Kosher Crunchy Dill Pickles	Vlasic	1 oz.	4
Kosher Dill Pickle Chips	generic	1 oz.	4
Kosher Dill Pickle Gherkins	Vlasic	1 oz.	4
Kosher Dill Pickle Spears	Vlasic	1 oz.	4
Kosher Dill Pickle Spears	generic	1 oz.	4
Kosher Dill Pickles Spears (1/2 the salt)	Vlasic	1 oz.	4
Kosher Dill Pickles	generic	1 piece	9
Kosher Pickle Halves	generic	1 piece	9
Kosher Pickle Slices	generic	1 oz.	3
Kosher Pickles	generic	2 oz.	7
Kosher Snack Pickle Chunks	Vlasic	1 oz.	4
Kosher Whole Pickles	generic	1 oz.	2
Lemon & Herb	Mrs. Dash (spice blends)	1 tsp.	12

Control your food. Do not be controlled by food.

Condiments

Product	Manufacturer	Serving Size	Calories
Lemon Extract	Durkee	1 tsp.	17
Lemon Extract, Cold	McCormick/Schilling	1 tsp.	35
Lemon Extract, Heated	McCormick/Schilling	1 tsp.	1
Lemon Pepper	Lawry's (Spice Blends)	1 tsp.	6
Lemon Pepper	McCormick/Schilling (spice blends)	1 tsp.	15
Lemon Pepper Seafood Seasoning	Golden Dipt	1/4 tsp.	8
Low Calorie Sweetener	Sweet 'N Low	1 pack	4
Low Pepper	Mrs. Dash (spice blends)	1 tsp.	12
Malt Extract, Dried	Durkee	1 oz.	104
Maple Extract	Durkee	1 tsp.	6
Maple-Imitation Flavor	McCormick/Schilling	1 tsp.	8
Maya Maize Popcorn	Nile Spice (spice blends)	1/2 tsp.	0
Medium Picante Sauce	Guiltless Gourmet	1 oz.	6
Mexican Shaker	Diamond Crystal	1/2 tsp.	4
Mild Pinto Bean Dip	Guiltless Gourmet	1 oz.	25
Mild Salsa	Guiltless Gourmet	1 oz.	6
Mild Salsa	Newman's Own	2 Tbsp.	10
Minced Onion	Lawry's (Spice Blends)	1 tsp.	7
Mint & Peppermint Pure Extract	McCormick/Schilling	1 tsp.	20

Find ways to walk and stretch daily.

Condiments

Product	Manufacturer	Serving Size	Calories
Molasses, Light	Brer Rabbit	2 Tbsp.	110
Nile Spice	Nile Spice (spice blends)	1/8 tsp.	0
No Garlic	Mrs. Dash (spice blends)	1 tsp.	12
Non Fat Tartar Sauce	Kraft	1 Tbsp.	10
Old Fashioned Dark Brown Sugar	Domino	1 tsp.	16
Old Fashioned Kosher Pickle Chips	generic	1 oz.	4
Old Fashioned Kosher Pickle Halves	generic	1 oz.	4
Old Fashioned Whole Kosher Pickles	generic	1 oz.	4
Orange Extract	Durkee	1 tsp.	14
Orange Pure Extract	McCormick/ Schilling	1 tsp.	23
Oriental Sweet and Sour Sauce	Bennett's	1 Tbsp.	30
Original	Mrs. Dash (spice blends)	1 tsp.	12
Original Dill Pickle	Vlasic	1 oz.	2
Original New Barbecue Sauce	Healthy Choice	2 Tbsp.	30
Original Syrup, maple taste	Aunt Jemima	1 fl. oz.	100
Peppermint Extract	Durkee	1 tsp.	15
Picalilli Pickles	generic	1 oz.	30
Picante Sauce	Wise	2 Tbsp.	12
Pickled Cucumbers	generic	2 spears	13
Pineapple Flavor	Durkee	1 tsp.	6
Pineapple-Imitation Extract	McCormick/ Schilling	1 tsp.	12

Choose a cereal with at least four grams of fiber per one ounce serving.

Condiments

Product	Manufacturer	Serving Size	Calories
Polish Snack Pickle Chunks (original)	Vlasic	1 oz.	4
Polish style Dill pickle spears	generic	1 oz.	4
Polish style dill pickles	generic	1 oz.	4
Popcorn Blend	McCormick/Schilling (spice blends)	1 tsp.	10
Processed dill pickles	generic	1 oz.	2
Pure Cane Granulated Sugar	Domino	1 tsp.	16
Pure Cane Sugar	Domino	1/2 cup	240
Pure Cane Sugar Packets	Domino	1 pack	16
Raspberry Extract	Durkee	1 tsp.	10
Root Beer Concentrate	McCormick/ Schilling	1 tsp.	13
Rum Flavor	Durkee	1 tsp.	14
Rum - Imitation Extract	McCormick/ Schilling	1 tsp.	19
Salt-Free 17	Lawry's (Spice Blends)	1 tsp.	10
Seasoned Lite Salt	Lawry's (Spice Blends)	1 tsp.	8
Seasoned Pepper	Lawry's (Spice Blends)	1 tsp.	9
Seasoned Salt	Lawry's (Spice Blends)	1 tsp.	4
Seasoned Salt Free	Lawry's (Spice Blends)	1 tsp.	3
Seasoning of Garlic	Nile Spice (spice blends)	1/8 tsp.	0

Cereals can be stored, unopened, for up to
one year in a cool, dry place.

Condiments

Product	Manufacturer	Serving Size	Calories
Sherry-Pure Extract	McCormick/ Schilling	1 tsp.	14
Sour Pickles	generic	1 oz.	3
Spaghetti Sauce, Chunky Garlic & Onion	Healthy Choice	4 oz.	40
Spaghetti Sauce, Chunky Italian Style	Healthy Choice	4 oz.	45
Spicy Black Bean Dip	Guiltless Gourmet	1 oz.	25
Spicy Lemon Pepper	Nile Spice (spice blends)	1/8 tsp.	0
Spoonful Sweetener	Nutra Sweet	1 Tbsp.	2
Steak Sauce	A-1	1 Tbsp.	14
Steak Sauce	Estee	1/2 oz.	15
Steak Sauce	French's	1 Tbsp.	16
Strawberry Extract	Durkee	1 tsp.	12
Strawberry-Imitation Extract	McCormick/ Schilling	1 tsp.	7
Sugar Substitute	Staff	1 pack	4
Sweet & Sour Sauce	Kraft	2 Tbsp.	50
Sweet Butter Pickle Chips	Vlasic	1 oz.	30
Sweet Butter Pickle Chips (1/2 the salt)	Vlasic	1 oz.	30
Sweet Butter Pickle Sticks	Vlasic	1 oz.	18
Sweet Cucumber Pickle Slices	generic	1 oz.	20
Sweet Cucumber Pickle Sticks	generic	1 oz.	25
Sweet Gherkins Pickled	generic	1 oz.	35

Choose whole grain cereals, such as oatmeal, shredded wheat, and whole grain wheat, oat, and rice flakes.

Condiments

Product	Manufacturer	Serving Size	Calories
Sweet Midget Gherkins Pickled	generic	1 oz.	35
Sweet Mixed Pickles	generic	1 oz.	40
Sweet Pickle Slices	generic	1 oz.	35
Sweet Pickles	generic	1 oz.	35
Sweet Salad Cubes	generic	1 oz.	30
Sweetener, 50 packets	Equal	1 pk.	4
Syrup	Hungry Jack	2 Tbsp.	100
Syrup, Butter Lite	Aunt Jemima	2 Tbsp.	50
Syrup, Dark Corn	Karo	1 Tbsp.	60
Syrup, Light	Brer Rabbit	2 Tbsp.	120
Syrup, Lite	Log Cabin	2 Tbsp.	50
Syrup, Lite	Staff	2 Tbsp.	50
Syrup, Lite Apple Cinnamon	Knotts Berry Farm	1 fl. oz.	50
Syrup, Lite, Blueberry	Knotts Berry Farm	1 fl. oz.	50
Syrup, Lite, Corn	Karo	1 fl. oz.	60
Syrup, Lite, Country	Knotts Berry Farm	1 fl. oz.	45
Syrup, Maple Breakfast	Estee	1 Tbsp.	12
Syrup, Pancake	Karo	1 fl. oz.	60
Table Blend	Mrs. Dash (spice blends)	1 tsp.	9
Taco Sauce	Wise	2 Tbsp.	12
Taco Sauce, Red, Mild	El Molino	2 Tbsp.	10
Taco Sauce, Thick, Smooth, Hot	Ortega	1 Tbsp.	8

Spaghettini is thin, long, and round pasta.

Condiments

Product	Manufacturer	Serving Size	Calories
Taco Sauce, Thick, Smooth, Mild	Ortega	1 Tbsp.	8
Taco Sauce, Western Style	Ortega	1 Tbsp.	8
Thick & Chunky Salsa, Hot	Ortega	1 Tbsp.	4
Thick & Chunky Salsa, Med.	Ortega	1 Tbsp.	4
Thick & Chunky Salsa, Mild	Ortega	1 Tbsp.	4
Thick & Rich Cajun Sauce	Heinz	1 oz.	35
Thick & Rich Chunky Sauce	Heinz	1 oz.	30
Thick & Rich Hawaiian Sauce	Heinz	1 oz.	40
Thick & Rich Hickory Smoke Sauce	Heinz	1 oz.	35
Thick & Rich Mesquite Sauce	Heinz	1 oz.	30
Thick & Rich Old Fashioned Sauce	Heinz	1 oz.	35
Thick & Rich Onion Sauce	Heinz	1 oz.	30
Thick & Rich Original Sauce	Heinz	1 oz.	35
Thick & Rich Texas Hot Sauce	Heinz	1 oz.	30
Tomato Ketchup	Healthy Choice	1/2 oz.	10
Tomato Ketchup	Hunt's	1 Tbsp.	15
Vanilla Butter & Nut Extract	Durkee	1 tsp.	5

Spaghetti is long and round pasta.

Condiments

Product	Manufacturer	Serving Size	Calories
Vanilla Cold Extract	McCormick/ Schilling	1 tsp.	12
Vanilla Flavor	Durkee	1 tsp.	3
Vanilla Heated Extract	McCormick/ Schilling	1 tsp.	1
Vanilla Pure Extract	Durkee	1 tsp.	8
Western Style Barbecue Sauce	Staff	1 Tbsp.	30
Whole Dill Pickles	Featherweight	1 piece	4
Zesty Crunchy Dill Pickles (original)	Vlasic	1 oz.	4
Zesty Dill Pickle Snack Chunks (original)	Vlasic	1 oz.	4
Zesty Dill Pickle Spears (original)	Vlasic	1 oz.	4

Cut fruits and vegetables with a stainless steel knife to prevent
browning of the produce.

Dairy

Product	Manufacturer	Serving Size	Calories
Amaretto, FF, Creamer, no cholesterol	International Delight	1 Tbsp.	30
Cheddar Cheese, FF	Lifetime Natural	1 oz.	40
Cheese, FF, Mozzarella, shredded	Healthy Choice	1 oz.	290
Cheese Spread, Free-N-Lean	Alpine Lace	1 oz.	30
Cheese Spread, Free-N-Lean, with Jalapeno	Alpine Lace	1 oz.	30
Cheese, FF, Singles, Swiss	Kraft	1 oz.	45
Cheese, FF, Swiss	Borden	1 oz.	40
Cheese, FF	Healthy Choice	1 oz.	210
Cheese, FF, fancy, shredded	Healthy Choice	1 oz.	310
Cheese, FF, Herb & Garlic	Healthy Choice	1 oz.	310
Cheese, FF, Mozzarella, shredded	Healthy Choice	1 oz.	290
Cheese, FF, Singles	Borden	1 oz.	40
Cheese, FF, Singles	Kraft	1 oz.	45
Cheese, Free-N-Lean, Natural	Alpine Lace	1 oz.	40
Cheese, Free-N-Lean, Cheddar	Alpine Lace	1 oz.	35
Cheese, Free-N-Lean Past. Process American	Alpine Lace	1 oz.	40

To retain vitamins when cooking vegetables, steaming and microwaving are the best methods.

Dairy

Product	Manufacturer	Serving Size	Calories
Cheese, Free-N-Lean, Past. Process Mozzarella	Alpine Lace	1 oz.	40
Cheese, Lite Line, FF, Sharp	Borden	1 slice	25
Cheese, Lite Line, FF, Singles	Borden	1 slice	25
Cheese, Lite, FF, Ricotta, Tub	Frigo	1 oz.	20
Cream, imitation, (veg. fat), whipped topping	generic	1 Tbsp.	10
Dry Milk powder, non-fat	generic	1 cup	255
Egg Beaters	Fleischmann's	1/4 cup	25
Egg Substitution	Healthy Choice	1/2 cup	30
Egg Whites, hard boiled	generic	1 large egg	15
Eggs, large, raw, white	generic	1 egg	15
FF, Creme Cheese	Alpine Lace	1 oz.	30
FF, Creme Cheese Block	Healthy Choice	1 oz.	30
FF, Singles Sharp Cheddar	Kraft	1 oz.	45
FF, Singles Swiss	Kraft	1 oz.	45
FF, Swiss Cheese	Borden	1 slice	30
Free N' Leen Cheddar	Alpine Lace	1 oz.	40
Free N' Leen Cheddar, grated	Alpine Lace	1 oz.	40
Free N' Leen Mozzarella	Alpine Lace	1 oz.	35
Free N' Lean Singles	Alpine Lace	1 oz.	40
French Vanilla Royal, FF, Creamer	International Delight	1 Tbsp.	30

Pears should be clean, firm, and bright.

Dairy

Product	Manufacturer	Serving Size	Calories
Hawaiian Macadamia, FF, Creamer	International Delight	1 Tbsp.	30
Irish Creme, FF, Creamer	International Delight	1 Tbsp.	30
Jack Cheese, FF	Lifetime Natural	1 oz.	40
Non Fat Cheese Slices	Weight Watchers	1 slice	25
Philadelphia Cream Cheese, FF, tub	Kraft	1 oz.	25
Philadelphia Cream Cheese, Free, non-fat	Kraft	1 oz.	25

Avoid rock-hard mangoes – they may not ripen properly.
Choose plump and firm fruit with clean color.

Dressings and Spreads

Product	Manufacturer	Serving Size	Calories
100% Pure Fruit Spreads, Apple	Poiret	1/2 tsp.	17
100% Pure Fruit Spreads, Pear-Apricot-Apple	Poiret	1/2 tsp.	17
100% Pure Fruit Spreads, Pear-Black Cherry	Poiret	1/2 oz.	35
100% Pure Fruit Spreads, Pear-Strawberry	Poiret	1/2 oz.	35
100% Pure Fruit Spreads, Pear-Strawberry	Poiret	1/2 tsp.	17
100% Spreadable Fruit, Apricot	Sorrell Ridge	1 tsp.	13
100% Spreadable Fruit, Boysenberry	Sorrell Ridge	1 tsp.	13
100% Spreadable Fruit, Raspberry	Sorrell Ridge	1 tsp.	13
100% Spreadable Fruit, Strawberry	Sorrell Ridge	1 tsp.	13
All fruit spread	generic	1 tsp.	8
All Fruit Spread, Apricot	Polaner	1/2 tsp.	17
All Fruit Spread, Black Cherry	Polaner	1 tsp.	14
All Fruit Spread, Blackberry	Polaner	1 tsp.	14
All Fruit Spread, Blueberry	Polaner	1 tsp.	14
All Fruit Spread, Raspberry	Polaner	1 tsp.	14

Lemons and limes should have firm, smooth skins.

Dressings and Spreads

Product	Manufacturer	Serving Size	Calories
All Fruit Spread, Strawberry	Polaner	1 tsp.	14
Apple Butter Spread	Bama	2 tsp.	25
Apple Butter Spread	White House	1 oz.	50
Apple Butter, Autumn Harvest Spread	Smucker's	1 oz.	50
Apple Butter, Natural Spread	Smucker's	1 tsp.	12
Apple Butter, Simply Fruit Spread	Smucker's	1 tsp.	12
Apple Cider Butter Spread	Smucker's	1 tsp.	12
Apple fruit spread	generic	1 tsp.	8
Apricot fruit spread	generic	1 tsp.	16
Canola Oil Cooking and Baking Spray	Staff	.25 g	0
Cheese Fantastic Spread	Bernsteins Light Fantastic	1 Tbsp.	14
Classico Italian Spread	Bernsteins Light Fantastic	1 Tbsp.	18
Cooking spray	generic	1 spray	2
FF, mayonnaise	generic	1 cup	192
Fruit Spread Light, Apricot & Pineapple	Knott's Berry Farm	1 tsp.	8
Fruit Spread, Blueberry	Pritikin	1 tsp.	14
Fruit Spread, Light, Apricot	Smucker's	1 tsp.	7
Fruit Spread, Light, Blackberry	Knott's Berry Farm	1 tsp.	8
Fruit Spread, Light, Boysenberry	Knott's Berry Farm	1 tsp.	8

Find kiwi fruit that is firm, but slightly soft to the touch when ripe.
Avoid bruised, soft, or moldy fruit.

Dressings and Spreads

Product	Manufacturer	Serving Size	Calories
Fruit Spread, Light, Concord Grape	Knott's Berry Farm	1 tsp.	8
Fruit Spread, Light, Orange Marmalade	Smucker's	1 tsp.	7
Fruit Spread, Light, Raspberry & Cranberry	Knott's Berry Farm	1 tsp.	8
Fruit Spread, Light, Red Raspberry	Smucker's	1 tsp.	7
Jam, Blackberry, seedless	Mary Ellen	2 tsp.	35
Jam, Blackberry, sugar free	Nutradiet	1 tsp.	4
Jam, Blueberry, reduced calorie	S + W	1 tsp.	4
Jam, Cherry	Bama	3.5 oz.	250
Jam, Concord Grape	Empress	2 tsp.	35
Jam, Grape	Empress	2 tsp.	35
Jam, Grape	Mary Ellen	2 tsp.	35
Jam, Orange	Bama	3.5 oz.	243
Jam, Plum	Bama	3.5 oz.	241
Jam, Quince	Bama	3.5 oz.	236
Jam, Raspberry	Bama	3.5 oz.	248
Jam, Red Cherry	Country Pure	2 tsp.	35
Jam, Red Current	Bama	3.5 oz.	237
Jam, Red Plum	Bama	2 tsp.	30
Jam, Red Raspberry	Country Pure	2 tsp.	35
Jam, Red Raspberry	Mary Ellen	2 tsp.	35
Jam, Red Raspberry	S & W	1 tsp.	4
Jam, Red Raspberry, sugar free	Nutradiet	1 tsp.	4

Grapes should be firm, ripe, and colorful in full bunches.
They should be firmly attached to the stem.

Dressings and Spreads

Product	Manufacturer	Serving Size	Calories
Jam, Simply Fruit, Apricot	Smucker's	1 tsp.	16
Jam, Simply Fruit, Blueberry	Smucker's	1 tsp.	16
Jam, Strawberry	Bama	3.5 oz.	234
Jam, Strawberry	Country Pure	2 tsp.	35
Jam, Strawberry	Mary Ellen	2 tsp.	35
Jam, Strawberry	S & W	1 tsp.	4
Jam, Strawberry sugar free	Nutradiet	1 tsp.	4
Jelly, All Varieties	Kraft	1 tsp.	17
Jelly, Apple	Bama	2 tsp.	30
Jelly, Apple	Bama	3.5 oz.	259
Jelly, Apple	Empress	2 tsp.	35
Jelly, Blackberry	Empress	2 tsp.	35
Jelly, Concord Grape, reduced calorie	S & W	1 tsp.	4
Jelly, Concord Grape, sugar free	Nutradiet	1 tsp.	4
Jelly, Grape	Bama	2 tsp.	30
Jelly, Grape	Mary Ellen	2 tsp.	35
Jelly, Grape, reduced calorie	Kraft	1 tsp.	6
Jelly, Imitation Blackberry, reduced calorie	Smucker's	3/8 oz.	4
Jelly, Imitation Cherry, reduced calorie	Smucker's	3/8 oz.	4
Jelly, Imitation Grape, reduced calorie	Smucker's	3/8 oz.	4

Hazelnut oil has a dark, amber color
with a nutty, smoky flavor.

Dressings and Spreads

Product	Manufacturer	Serving Size	Calories
Jelly, Mixed Fruit	Empress	2 tsp.	35
Jelly, Orange Marmalade, sugar free	Nutradiet	1 tsp.	4
Jelly, Raspberry	Bama	3.5 oz.	259
Jelly, Red Current	Empress	2 tsp.	35
Jelly, Red Current	Bama	3.5 oz.	265
Jelly, Rose Hip	Bama	3.5 oz.	250
Jelly, Single Serving (all flavors)	Smucker's	1/2 oz.	38
Jelly, Strawberry	Mary Ellen	2 tsp.	35
Kraft Free, Mayonnaise	Kraft	1 Tbsp.	8
Kraft Free, Miracle Whip	Kraft	1 Tbsp.	15
Lite Fruit Spread, Apricot & Pineapple	Knott's Berry Farm	1 Tbsp.	8
Lite Fruit Spread, Blackberry	Knott's Berry Farm	1 Tbsp.	8
Lite Fruit Spread, Boysenberry	Knott's Berry Farm	1 Tbsp.	8
Lite Fruit Spread, Concord Grape	Knott's Berry Farm	1 Tbsp.	8
Lite Fruit Spread, Raspberry & Cranberry	Knott's Berry Farm	1 Tbsp.	8
Low Sugar Grape Fruit Spread	Bama	1 tsp.	8
Low Sugar Peach Fruit Spread	Bama	1 tsp.	8
Low Sugar Strawberry Fruit Spread	Bama	1 tsp.	8
Marmalade, California Orange	Empress	2 tsp.	35
Orange Marmalade	S & W	1 tsp.	4

Cottonseed oil possesses a bland flavor
and a pale yellow color.

Dressings and Salads

Product	Manufacturer	Serving Size	Calories
Peach Butter Spread	Smucker's	1 tsp.	15
Peach Fruit Spread	Pritikin	1 tsp.	14
Preserves, All Flavors	Smucker's	1 tsp.	18
Preserves, All Varieties	Kraft	1 tsp.	17
Preserves, Apricot	Empress	2 tsp.	35
Preserves, Apricot Pineapple	Empress	2 tsp.	35
Preserves, Apricot-Pineapple, sugar free	Nutradiet	1 tsp.	4
Preserves, Black Cherry	Empress	2 tsp.	35
Preserves, Black Raspberry	Empress	2 tsp.	35
Preserves, Boysenberry	Empress	2 tsp.	35
Preserves, Boysenberry, sugar free	Nutradiet	1 tsp.	4
Preserves, Natural Strawberry	Bama	1 tsp.	16
Preserves, Peach	Bama	2 tsp.	30
Preserves, Peach	Empress	2 tsp.	35
Preserves, Peach Pineapple	Empress	2 tsp.	35
Preserves, Plum	Empress	2 tsp.	35
Preserves, Red Cherry	Empress	2 tsp.	35
Preserves, Red Raspberry	Empress	2 tsp.	35
Preserves, Red Tart Cherry	S & W	1 tsp.	4
Preserves, Seedless Blackberry	Empress	2 tsp.	35

Corn oil is golden in color with a mild flavor.

Dressings and Spreads

Product	Manufacturer	Serving Size	Calories
Preserves, Single Serving (all flavors)	Smucker's	1/2 oz.	38
Preserves, Strawberry	Empress	2 tsp.	35
Red Raspberry Fruit Spread	Pritikin	1 tsp.	14
Red Wine Vinegar	Seven Seas Free	1 Tbsp.	6
Salad Dressing FF, Italian	Pfeifer Foods	1 Tbsp.	5
Salad Dressing FF, Ranch	Pfeifer Foods	1 Tbsp.	15
Salad Dressing, Blue Cheese FF	Kraft Free	1 Tbsp.	16
Salad Dressing, Blue Cheese low calorie	Estee	1 Tbsp.	8
Salad Dressing, Catalina Free	Kraft	1 Tbsp.	18
Salad Dressing, Caesar	Weight Watchers	1 Tbsp.	4
Salad Dressing, Caesar	Weight Watchers	1 pouch	6
Salad Dressing, Chunky Blue Cheese	Wish Bone	5 oz.	0
Salad Dressing, Creamy Cucumber	Weight Watchers	1 Tbsp.	18
Salad Dressing, Creamy Dijon	Bernsteins Light Fantastic	1 Tbsp.	20
Salad Dressing, Creamy French	Estee	1 Tbsp.	6
Salad Dressing, Creamy Garlic, reduced calorie	Estee	1 Tbsp.	2

Canola oil has a light yellow color and a bland flavor.

Dressings and Spreads

Product	Manufacturer	Serving Size	Calories
Salad Dressing, Creamy Italian	Weight Watchers	1 Tbsp.	12
Salad Dressing, Cream Italian, reduced calorie	Estee	1 Tbsp.	6
Salad Dressing, Creamy Peppercorn	Weight Watchers	1 Tbsp.	8
Salad Dressing, Creamy Ranch	Weight Watchers	1 Tbsp.	25
Salad Dressing, Creamy Ranch	Weight Watchers	1 pouch	35
Salad Dressing, FF, Italian	Astor	1 Tbsp.	5
Salad Dressing, FF, Thousand Island	Astor	1 Tbsp.	15
Salad Dressing, FF, Blue Cheese	Walden Farm's	1 Tbsp.	10
Salad Dressing, FF, Caesar	Walden Farm's	1 Tbsp.	10
Salad Dressing, FF, Creamy Italian	Walden Farm's	1 Tbsp.	10
Salad Dressing, FF, French	Walden Farm's	1 Tbsp.	10
Salad Dressing, FF, Honey Dijon	Walden Farm's	1 Tbsp.	10
Salad Dressing, FF, Italian	Walden Farm's	1 Tbsp.	10
Salad Dressing, FF Italian, Sodium Free	Walden Farm's	1 Tbsp.	10
Salad Dressing, FF, Mayo Style	Weight Watchers	1 Tbsp.	12

Viennese coffee is a strong, hot coffee steeped with spices, strained into cups, and served with whipped cream.

Dressings and Spreads

Product	Manufacturer	Serving Size	Calories
Salad Dressing, FF, Ranch	Walden Farm's	1 Tbsp.	10
Salad Dressing, FF, Russian	Walden Farm's	1 Tbsp.	10
Salad Dressing, FF, Whipped	Weight Watchers	1 Tbsp.	10
Salad Dressing, FF, Zesty Classic Herb	Walden Farm's	1 Tbsp.	10
Salad Dressing, FF, Zesty Italian Vinagrette	Walden Farm's	1 Tbsp.	10
Salad Dressing, Free, Italian	Seven Seas	1 Tbsp.	4
Salad Dressing, French Free	Kraft	1 Tbsp.	20
Salad Dressing, French Style	Pritikin	1 Tbsp.	10
Salad Dressing, French Style	Weight Watchers	1 Tbsp.	10
Salad Dressing, Honey Dijon	Healthy Sensations	1 Tbsp.	25
Salad Dressing, Honey Dijon Free	Kraft	1 Tbsp.	20
Salad Dressing, Italian	Pritikin	1 Tbsp.	8
Salad dressing, Italian	generic	1 cup	64
Salad Dressing, Italian, FF	Healthy Sensations	1 Tbsp.	7
Salad Dressing, Italian Mix, no oil	Good Seasons	1 packet	112
Salad Dressing, Italian, no oil	Good	1 Tbsp.	7
Salad Dressing, Italian Style	Weight Watchers	1 Tbsp.	6

Irish coffee is a mix of hot coffee and Irish whiskey,
topped with whipped cream.

Dressings and Spreads

Product	Manufacturer	Serving Size	Calories
Salad Dressing, Italian with Sun-Dried Tomatoes	Walden Farm's	1 Tbsp.	9
Salad Dressing, Kraft Free, Peppercorn	Kraft	1 Tbsp.	18
Salad Dressing, Kraft Free, Ranch	Kraft	1 Tbsp.	20
Salad Dressing, Kraft Free, Thousand Island	Kraft	1 Tbsp.	20
Salad Dressing, Kraft, Oil Free Italian	Kraft	1 Tbsp.	4
Salad Dressing, Kraft Free, Italian	Kraft	1 Tbsp.	4
Salad Dressing, Lite, Italian	Wish Bone	.5 oz.	6
Salad Dressing, Ranch	Pritikin	1 Tbsp.	16
Salad Dressing, Ranch	Seven Seas Free	1 Tbsp.	16
Salad Dressing, Russian	Pritikin	1 Tbsp.	12
Salad Dressing, Thousand Island	Walden Farm's	1 Tbsp.	10
Salad Dressing, Zesty Italian, reduced calorie	Estee	1 Tbsp.	2
Sauce, Butterscotch, sugar free	Steel's	1/2 oz.	39.96
Sauce, Red Raspberry, sugar free	Steel's	1/2 oz.	23
Simply Fruit Spread, all flavors	Smucker's	1 tsp.	10
Simply Fruit, Orange Marmalade Spread	Smucker's	1 tsp.	18

Mocha java is a mix of regular, straight coffee and hot cocoa.

Dressings and Spreads

Product	Manufacturer	Serving Size	Calories
Spread, low sugar, Apricot	Smucker's	1 tsp.	8
Spread, low sugar, All Flavors	Smucker's	1 tsp.	8
Spread, low sugar, Orange Marmalade	Smucker's	1 tsp.	8
Spread, low sugar, Red Raspberry	Smucker's	1 tsp.	8
Spread, low sugar, Strawberry	Smucker's	1 tsp.	8
Spread, Pumpkin Butter, Autumn Harvest	Smucker's	1 tsp.	12
Strawberry Fruit Spread	Pritikin	1 tsp.	14
Toppings, Strawberry	Smucker's	2 Tbsp.	120
Totally Fruit, Spreadable, Apricot	Welch's	1 tsp.	14
Totally Fruit, Spreadable, Strawberry	Welch's	1 tsp.	14
Vanilla, Nature Sweet Sugar-Free Sweetener	Steel's	1/2 oz.	23
Veg. Cooking and Baking Spray	Staff	.25 g	0

Demitasse is a strong coffee, made from a dark roast.

Fruits

Product	Manufacturer	Serving Size	Calories
Apple Chunk's	Sunmaid Sunsweet	1/2 cup	150
Apple, golden delicious	generic	1 apple	80
Apple, Sliced	Del Monte	1/4 cup	140
Applesauce, Chunky, Natural	Mott's	1/2 cup	82
Applesauce, chunky, natural	Mott's	1/2 cup	82
Applesauce, Lite Fruit's	Del Monte	1/2 cup	50
Applesauce, unsweetened	Luckey Leaf	1/2 cup	50
Applesauce, unsweetened	Stokely	1/2 cup	45
Apricot Halves, Lite Fruit's	Del Monte	1/2 cup	60
Apricots, canned fruit, heavy syrup	generic	1 cup	215
Apricots, raw w/o pits	generic	3 apricots	50
Bite-Size Pitted Prunes	Sunsweet	2 oz.	140
Blueberries, frozen, sweetened	generic	10 oz.	130
Breakfast Prunes	Sunsweet	2 oz.	120
California Golden Raisins	Sun-Maid	1/4 cup	250
California Seedless Raisins, Mini-Snacks	Staff	1/4 cup	130
California Sun-Dried Raisins	Sun-Maid	1/4 cup	130
California Sun-Dried Raisins, 14 Mini-Snacks	Sun-Maid	1 box	45

Espresso, or expresso, is strong, dark coffee

Fruits

Product	Manufacturer	Serving Size	Calories
Cherries, sour, red	generic	1 cup	90
Chunky Mix, Lite Fruit's	Del Monte	1/2 cup	50
Chunky Mix, Lite Fruit's	Libby	1/2 cup	50
Chunky Mixed Fruit, diet	S + W	1/2 cup	40
Chunky Mixed Fruit, natural style	S + W	1/2 cup	90
Chunky Mixed Fruit, unsweetened	S + W	1/2 cup	40
Chunky Mixed Fruits, heavy syrup	Libby	1/2 cup	90
Chunky Pineapple, in juice	Del Monte	1/2 cup	70
Cranberries, raw	generic	1 cup	46
Cranberry Sauce, jellied	Ocean Spray	2 oz.	90
Cranberry Sauce, Old Fashioned	S & W	1/2 cup	90
Cranberry Sauce, whole berry	S & W	1/2 cup	90
Cranicot	Ocean Spray	6 oz.	110
Crushed Pineapple, in heavy syrup	Del Monte	1/2 cup	90
Crushed Pineapple, in heavy syrup	Dole	1/2 cup	90
Crushed Pineapple, in heavy syrup	Staff	1/2 cup	90
Crushed Pineapple, in juice	Del Monte	1/2 cup	70

Cafe au Lait is one-half strong coffee
and one-half hot milk.

Fruits

Product	Manufacturer	Serving Size	Calories
Crushed Pineapple, in juice	Staff	1/2 cup	70
Dates, chopped	Dromedary	1/4 cup	130
Dates, pitted and chopped	Dole	1/4 cup	140
Dates, whole, w/o pits	generic	10 dates	230
Dried Mixed Fruit	Del Monte	2 oz.	130
Fruit Cocktail (in heavy syrup)	Del Monte	1/2 cup	90
Fruit Cocktail (in heavy syrup)	Libby's	1/2 cup	90
Fruit Cocktail (in heavy syrup)	S & W	1/2 cup	90
Fruit Cocktail (in water)	Libby's	1/2 cup	40
Fruit Cocktail, Diet	S & W	1/2 cup	40
Fruit Cocktail, Natural Lite	S & W	1/2 cup	60
Fruit Cocktail, Natural Style	S & W	1/2 cup	40
Fruit Natural's (in its own juice)	Del Monte	1/2 cup	60
Grapes	generic	10 grapes	40
Grapefruit	generic	1/2 grapefruit	40
Grapefruit, canned, sections with syrup	generic	1 cup	150
Green Apples, chopped	generic	1 cup	65
Kiwifruit, raw	generic	1 kiwifruit	45
Large Prunes	Del Monte	2 oz.	120
Lemon	generic	1 lemon	17

Flavor is lost through evaporation, so don't overcook
your soups or vegetables.

Fruits

Product	Manufacturer	Serving Size	Calories
Lemon Essence Pitted Prunes	Sunsweet	6 prunes	100
Lime, slices/wedges	generic	1 lime	20
Lite Bartlett Pear Halves, (in ex-lite syrup)	Del Monte	1/2 cup	50
Lite Chunky Mixed Fruit (in syrup)	Del Monte	1/2 cup	50
Lite Fruit Cocktail (in ex-lite syrup)	Del Monte	1/2 cup	50
Lite Sliced Peaches (in ex-lite syrup)	Del Monte	1/2 cup	50
Mandarin Oranges	generic	1 cup	85
Medium Prunes	Del Monte	2 oz.	120
Melon, raw	generic	1/10 melon	45
Mixed Fruit, dried	Del Monte	1/4 cup	130
Mixed Fruit, Quick Thaw	Bird's Eye	1/2 cup	96
Natural Lite Apricot Halves (unpeeled)	Libby's	1/2 cup	60
Natural Lite Cocktail (in juice)	Libby's	1/2 cup	50
Natural Lite Pear Halves (in juice)	Libby's	1/2 cup	50
Natural Lite Sliced Peaches	Libby's	1/2 cup	50
Natural Lite Sliced Peaches (in juice)	Libby's	1/2 cup	50
Orange Essence Pitted Prunes	Sunsweet	6 prunes	100
Oranges, raw, whole	generic	1 orange	60
Oranges, Mandarin	Empress	5.5 oz.	100

Peel vegetables as thinly as possible to preserve the nutrients.
They are chiefly located just under the skin.

Fruits

Product	Manufacturer	Serving Size	Calories
Peaches, dried uncooked	Del Monte	1/4 cup	140
Peaches, dried uncooked	Sunmaid/ Sunsweet	1/4 cup	140
Peaches, raw, whole, peeled	generic	1 peach	35
Pear Halves (in heavy syrup)	Del Monte	1/2 cup	90
Pears, Lite Fruit's	Del Monte	1/2 cup	50
Pears, Lite Fruit's	Libby's	1/2 cup	60
Pineapple Chunks (in juice)	Dole	1/2 cup	70
Pineapple Slices (in heavy syrup)	Dole	2 slices	90
Pineapple Slices (in pineapple juice)	Dole	2 slices	70
Pineapple Chunks (in juice)	Staff	1/2 cup	70
Pineapple Tid Bit (in juice)	Del Monte	1/2 cup	70
Pineapple Tid Bits (in juice)	Dole	1/2 cup	70
Pineapple Wedges (in juice)	Del Monte	1/2 cup	70
Pitted Prunes	Del Monte	2 oz.	120
Pitted Prunes	Sunsweet	6 prunes	100
Plantains, w/o peel, cooked, boiled, sliced	generic	1 cup	180
Plums, w/o pits, canned, cooked, fruit & liquid	generic	3 plums	120

To restore color to fruits, mix 3 parts water with 1 part citrus (orange or lemon) juice, and rinse the fruit briefly in the mixture.

Fruits

Product	Manufacturer	Serving Size	Calories
Premium Apples	Mariani	1/4 cup	150
Premium Mediterranean Apricots	Mariani	1/4 cup	140
Premium Peaches	Mariani	1/4 cup	140
Premium Prunes, lg.	Mariani	2 oz.	140
Raspberries, light syrup, quick thaw	Bird's Eye	1/2 cup	80
Sliced Peaches (in heavy syrup)	Del Monte	1/2 cup	90
Sliced Pineapple (in heavy syrup)	Del Monte	1/2 cup	90
Sliced Pineapple (in heavy syrup)	Staff	4 slices	190
Sliced Pineapple (in its own juice)	Del Monte	1/2 cup	90
Sliced Pineapple (in its own juice)	Staff	2 slices	70
Sliced Dried Apples	Del Monte	2 oz.	120
Spear Pineapple (in juice)	Del Monte	2 spears	50
Strawberries, lite syrup, quick thaw	Bird's Eye	1/2 cup	96
Sun-Dried Peaches	Del Monte	2 oz.	120
Tangerines, canned, light syrup	generic	1 cup	155
Tropical Fruit Salad (in lite syrup)	Del Monte	1/2 cup	90
Zante Currents	Sun-Maid	1/4 cup	130

Treat vegetables that discolor with an acid such as lemon juice,
or keep in water until needed.

Grains, Rice, and Beans

Product	Manufacturer	Serving Size	Calories
Barbecue Pork Recipe	Shake 'n Bake	1/8 pouch	35
Beans, FF, Fast Menu, Amaranth	Health Valley	5 oz.	70
Beans, FF, Fast Menu, Hearty Lentil	Health Valley	5 oz.	80
Beans, FF, Fast Menu, Black Bean	Health Valley	5 oz.	70
Brava, Re-Fried Beans	La Victoria	1 Tbsp.	6
Brown rice, raw	generic	1 cup	540
Casera Re-Fried Beans	La Victoria	1 Tbsp.	4
Chicken Flavor Rice Pilaf Mix	Near East	1 oz.	120
Corn Cakes, Nacho	Quaker	1 cake	40
Corn Flake Crumbs	Kellogg's	1 oz.	100
Couscous Moroccan Pasta	Near East	1/4 oz.	150
Coutettes Stuffing Mix	Kellogg's	1 oz.	100
Green Chili Re-Fried Beans	La Victoria	1 Tbsp.	3
Green Jalapeno Re-Fried Beans	La Victoria	1 Tbsp.	4
Honey Baked Beans, FF, no salt	Health Valley	5 oz.	100
Honey Baked Beans, FF, with salt	Health Valley	5 oz.	100
Lentil Pilaf Mix	Near East	1 oz.	130
Long Grain & Wild Rice	Near East	1 oz.	120

Buy a firm head of cabbage with finely ribbed, crisp leaves.

Grains, Rice, and Beans

Product	Manufacturer	Serving Size	Calories
Long Grain & Wild Rice	Uncle Ben's	1/2 cup	100
Macaroni, cooked	generic	1 cup	115
Mini-Bagel	generic	1 bagel	70
Pasta, cooked	generic	1 cup	155
Popcorn Cakes, Butter Flavor	Quaker	1 cake	35
Popcorn Cakes, Lightly Salted	Quaker	1 cake	35
Popcorn Cakes, Mild White Cheddar	Quaker	1 cake	40
Rice Cakes, Apple Cinnamon	Quaker	1 cake	40
Rice Cakes, Mini, Apple Cinnamon	Hain	1/2 oz.	60
Rice Cakes, Mini, Plain	Hain	1/2 oz.	60
Rice Cakes, Mini, Teriyaki	Hain	1/2 oz.	50
Rice Pilaf Mix	Near East	1 oz.	120
Snack Cakes, no sodium	Quaker	1 cake	35
Snack Cakes, Rice Cake	Quaker	1 cake	35
Snack Cakes, Rye	Quaker	1 cake	35
Snack Cakes, Sesame	Quaker	1 cake	35
Snack Cakes, Wheat	Quaker	1 cake	35
Spanish Rice Mix	Near East	1 oz.	130
Taboule Wheat Salad Mix	Near East	3/4 oz.	100
Wheat Pilaf Mix	Near East	1 oz.	120

Find mushrooms with firm, white caps,
closed at the stem.

Juices

Product	Manufacturer	Serving Size	Calories
Juice, Apple	Bright + Early	8 fl. oz.	120
Juice, Apple	Indian Summer	6 fl. oz.	90
Juice, Apple	Staff	6 fl. oz.	90
Juice, Apple 100% Pure	Red Creek	6 fl. oz.	97
Juice, Apple Bowl	Campbell's	6 fl. oz.	110
Juice, Apple Cox's Orange Pippin	President's Choice	6 fl. oz.	90
Juice, Apple Frozen	Bird's Eye	6 fl. oz.	80
Juice, Apple Natural Style	Mott's	6 fl. oz.	88
Juice, Apple Natural Style	Red Creek	6 fl. oz.	97
Juice, Apple Sparkling	Martinelli's	6 fl. oz.	100
Juice, Apple Unsweetened	IGA	6 fl. oz.	74
Juice, Apple-Cranberry	Smucker's	8 fl. oz.	120
Juice, Apple-Cranberry Cocktail	Seneca	6 fl. oz.	110
Juice, Calypso Breeze Fruit	Chiquita	6 fl. oz.	100
Juice, Caribbean Splash Fruit	Chiquita	6 fl. oz.	90
Juice, Cocktail Vegetable canned	generic	1 cup	45
Juice, Cocktail 100% Grapefruit	Ocean Spray	6 fl. oz.	70
Juice, Cranberry Cocktail	Ocean Spray	6 fl. oz.	100

Look for firm, springy heads of lettuce that give slightly under gentle pressure.

Juices

Product	Manufacturer	Serving Size	Calories
Juice, Fruit Juicy Red	Hawaiian	6 fl. oz.	90
Juice, Grape	Staff	6 fl. oz.	90
Juice, Grape	Welch's Orchard	6 fl. oz.	130
Juice, Grape, fzn.	generic	1 cup	90
Juice, Grape-Apple	Welch's Orchard	6 fl. oz.	110
Juice, Grapefruit Frozen	generic	1 cup	100
Juice, Juicy Juice Berry, canned	Libby's	6 fl. oz.	90
Juice, Juicy Juice Grape, canned	Libby's	6 fl. oz.	90
Juice, Juicy Juice Punch, canned	Libby's	6 fl. oz.	90
Juice, Juicy Juice Tropical, canned	Libby's	6 fl. oz.	110
Juice, Juicy Juice Cherry, canned	Libby's	6 fl. oz.	90
Juice, Lemon canned/bottled	Staff	2 Tbsp.	6
Juice, Lemon Fresh	generic	1 tsp.	133
Juice, Lime Fresh	generic	1 cup	65
Juice, Orange, canned, unsweetened	Staff	6 fl. oz.	90
Juice, Orange, fzn. concentrate	generic	1 cup	110
Juice, Orange-Pineapple-Apple	Welch's Orchard	6 fl. oz.	110
Juice, Pineapple unsweetened, canned	generic	1 cup	140

The skin of garlic may be white or pink.

Juices

Product	Manufacturer	Serving Size	Calories
Juice, Prune canned/bottled	Sunsweet	1 cup	120
Juice, Ruby Grapefruit, unsweetened	generic	1 cup	95
Juice, Spicy Hot Canned	Campbell's	6 fl. oz.	35
Juice, Tangerine canned, unsweetened	generic	1 cup	95
Juice, Tomato	generic	1 Tbsp.	2.5
Juice, Tomato, canned	Campbell's	1 cup	40
Juice, Tomato, canned	Hunts	1 cup	40
Juice, Tomato canned	Sacramento	1 cup	40
Juice, Tomato, canned	Staff	1 cup	40
Juice, Tomato unsalted	generic	1 cup	40
Juice, V8 100% Vegetable	Campbell's	6 fl. oz.	35
Juice, White Grapefruit	Welch's Orchard	6 fl. oz.	100
Juices To Go, Apple	Minute Maid	9.6 fl. oz.	145
Nectar, Apricot	Libby's	6 fl. oz.	120
Nectar, Apricot-Orange	Kern's	6 fl. oz.	110
Nectar, Apricot-Pineapple	S + W	6 fl. oz.	120
Nectar, Banana	Libby's	6 fl. oz.	120
Nectar, Banana-Pineapple	Kern's	6 fl. oz.	120
Nectar, Guava	Libby's	6 fl. oz.	120
Nectar, Passion Fruit Orange	Kern's	6 fl. oz.	100

Dried papaya comes in long finger-shaped slices.

Juices

Product	Manufacturer	Serving Size	Calories
Nectar, Passion Fruit Orange	Libby's	8 fl. oz.	150
Nectar, Peach	Libby's	6 fl. oz.	120
Nectar, Pear	Libby	6 fl. oz.	120
Nectar, Strawberry-Banana	Kern's	6 fl. oz.	100
Nectar, Strawberry-Banana	Libby	8 fl. oz.	150
Nectar, Strawberry-Banana	Libby	6 fl. oz.	120
Nectar, Tropical	Kern's	6 fl. oz.	112

Look for cucumbers that are firm, dark green, and well shaped.

Meats and Fish

Product	Manufacturer	Serving Size	Calories
Clam Juice	Doxsee	3 oz.	4
Clams, fancy, chopped	S + W	2 oz.	28
Clams, fancy, minced	S & W	2 oz.	28
Clams, whole baby chowder	S & W	2 oz.	33
Cod, Today's Catch	Van de Kamp's	5 oz.	110
Fishfries,country style, Alaska Pollock	generic	3.75 oz.	120
Fishfries, country style Cod	generic	3.75 oz.	120
Fishfries, raw, Cod, nordic cut	generic	4 oz.	70
Fishfries, raw, Cod rectangles	generic	4 oz.	70
Fishfries, raw, grade A English cut Cod	generic	4 oz.	70
Fishfries, Santa Fe style, Alaska Pollock	generic	3.75 oz.	120
Fishfries, Santa Fe style, Cod	generic	3.75 oz.	120
Fishfries, southern style, Alaska Pollock	generic	3.75 oz.	120
Haddock, English cut, glazed	generic	4 oz.	70
Haddock, Nordic cut	generic	4 oz.	70

Corn on the cob should have fresh, moist husks. It should not be dry. Tender and milky when punctured.

Snacks, Cookies, and Cakes

Product	Manufacturer	Serving Size	Calories
Carrot Cake	Entenmann's	1 slice	100
Cookies, FF, Chocolate Brownie	Entenmann's	2 cookies	80
Cookies, FF, Fruit Centers, Apple	Health Valley	1 each	80
Cookies, FF, Fruit Centers, Apricot	Health Valley	1 each	80
Cookies, FF, Fruit Centers, Date	Health Valley	1 each	80
Cookies, FF, Fruit Centers, Raisin Apple	Health Valley	1 each	80
Cookies, FF, Fruit Centers, Raspberry	Health Valley	1 each	80
Cookies, FF, Fruit Centers, Tropical	Health Valley	1 each	80
Cookies, FF, Fruit Chunks, Apple Raisin	Health Valley	3 each	85
Cookies, FF, Fruit Chunks, Apricot-Apple	Health Valley	3 each	85
Cookies, FF, Fruit Chunks, Banana-Spice	Health Valley	3 each	85
Cookies, FF, Fruit Chunks, Oatmeal-Raisin	Health Valley	3 each	85
Cookies, FF, Fruit Chunks, Raspberry-Apple	Health Valley	3 each	85
Cookies, FF, Fruit, Apple-Spice	Health Valley	3 each	80
Cookies, FF, Fruit, Apricot Delight	Health Valley	3 each	80
Cookies, FF, Fruit, Date Delight	Health Valley	3 each	80

Raisin are high in iron and minerals.

Snacks, Cookies, and Cakes

Product	Manufacturer	Serving Size	Calories
Cookies, FF, Fruit, Hawaiian Fruit	Health Valley	3 each	80
Cookies, FF, Fruit, Raisin-Oatmeal	Health Valley	3 each	80
Cookies, FF, Graham Animal, Cinnamon	Health Valley	1 oz.	90
Cookies, FF, Graham Animal, Honey-Oat	Health Valley	1 oz.	90
Cookies, FF, Graham Animal, Nat. Chocolate	Health Valley	1 oz.	90
Cookies, FF, Healthy Chips	Health Valley	3 each	80
Cookies, FF, Healthy Granola	Health Valley	3 each	75
Cookies, FF, Jumbos, Apple Raisin	Health Valley	1 each	80
Cookies, FF, Jumbos, Raspberry	Health Valley	1 each	80
Cookies, FF, Mini Fruit Center, Apple	Health Valley	2 each	90
Cookies, FF, Mini Fruit Center, Orange	Health Valley	2 each	90
Cookies, FF, Mini Fruit Center, Peach	Health Valley	2 each	90
Cookies, FF, Mini Fruit Center, Raspberry	Health Valley	2 each	90
Cookies, FF Mini Fruit Center, Strawberry	Health Valley	2 each	90
Cookies, FF, Oatmeal-Raisin	Entenmann's	2 each	80
Cookies, FF, Oatmeal/Chocolate Chip	Entenmann's	2 each	80

Carrots should be bright orange in color, crisp, and straight.

Snacks, Cookies, and Cakes

Product	Manufacturer	Serving Size	Calories
Corn Flake Crumbs	Kellogg's	1/4 cup	100
Corn Flakes	Kellogg's	1 oz.	100
Corn Pops	Kellogg's	1 oz.	110
Cracker Meal	Golden Dipt	1 oz.	100
Cracker Meal	Nabisco	1 oz.	50
Crackers	Goya	1 cracker	30
Crackers, FF, Organic Whole Wheat	Health Valley	1/2 oz.	45
Crackers, FF, Organic Whole Wheat, Cheese	Health Valley	1/2 oz.	45
Crackers, FF, Organic Whole Wheat, Herb	Health Valley	1/2 oz.	45
Crackers, FF, Organic Whole Wheat, Onion	Health Valley	1/2 oz.	45
Crackers, FF, Organic Whole Wheat, Veg.	Health Valley	1/2 oz.	45
Crackers, Organic Whole Wheat	Health Valley	1/2 oz.	45
Crispbread	Weight Watchers	2 pieces	30
Crispbread, Extra Thin	Ideal	3 oz.	48
Crispbread, Oatbread Thins	Ideal	2 oz.	50
English Water Crackers	North Castle	1 cracker	10
FF, Apple Cinnamon Mini Rice Cakes	Quaker	1/2 oz.	50
FF, Apple Cinnamon Rice Cakes	Quaker	10 grams	40
FF, Butter Popped Corn Cakes	Quaker	9 grams	35

Look for broccoli that is bright green with tightly closed buds.

Snacks, Cookies, and Cakes

Product	Manufacturer	Serving Size	Calories
FF, Caramel Corn Cakes	Quaker	13 grams	50
FF, Caramel Corn Mini Rice Cakes	Quaker	1/2 oz.	50
FF, Honey Nut Mini Rice Cakes	Quaker	5 mini rice cakes	50
FF, Mini Popcorn Rice Cakes, buttered	Hain Pure Food Co.	1/2 oz.	45
FF, Mini Popcorn Rice Cakes, lightly salted	Hain Pure Food Co.	1/2 oz.	60
FF, White Cheddar Popped Corn Cakes	Quaker	10 grams	40
FF, Apple Bars Chewy Fruit Cookies	Crackin' Good Bakers	1 bar	80
FF, Apple Buns	Entenmann's	1 bun	50
FF, Banana Loaf	Entenmann's	1.3 oz.	90
FF, Bavarian Creme Pastry	Entenmann's	1.3 oz.	80
FF, Blueberry Cheese Coffee Cake	Entenmann's	1 oz.	90
FF, Caramel Corn Puffs	Health Valley	1 oz.	100
FF, Caramel Corn Puffs, Original Style	Health Valley	1 oz.	100
FF, Caramel Corn Puffs, Peanut Flavor	Health Valley	1 oz.	100
FF, Cheese Flavored Puffs	Health Valley	1 oz.	100
FF, Cheese Flavored Puffs, with Chili	Health Valley	1 oz.	100

Shelled lima beans should be plump,
with tender skins.

Snacks, Cookies, and Cakes

Product	Manufacturer	Serving Size	Calories
FF, Cheese Flavored Puffs, with Green Onion	Health Valley	1 oz.	100
FF, Cinnamon Ring	Entenmann's	1 oz.	80
FF, Cranberry Orange Cake	Entenmann's	1 oz.	70
FF, Deli Style Original Bread Sticks	Stella D'oro	5 bread sticks	60
FF, Fig Bars Chewy Fruit Cookies	Crackin' Good Bakers	1 bar	75
FF, Fig Newtons	Nabisco	1 cookie	70
FF, Fig Newtons, Apple	Nabisco	1 cookie	70
FF, Fig Newtons, Cranberry	Nabisco	1 cookie	70
FF, Fig Newtons, Raspberry	Nabisco	1 cookie	70
FF, Fig Newtons, Strawberry	Nabisco	1 cookie	60
FF, Fruit Bars, Apple	Health Valley	1 bar	140
FF, Fruit Bars, Apricot	Health Valley	1 bar	140
FF, Fruit Bars, Date	Health Valley	1 bar	140
FF, Fruit Bars, Raisin	Health Valley	1 bar	140
FF, Fruit Delight Cookies Apple-Cinnamon	Stella D'oro	1 cookie	70
FF, Fruit Delight Cookies, Peach-Apricot	Stella D'oro	1 cookie	70
FF, Fruit Slices	Stella D'oro	1 cookie	50
FF, Fudge Iced Chocolate Cake	Entenmann's	1.3 oz.	90
FF, Granola Bars, Blueberry	Health Valley	1 bar	140

Currants are sweet and high in iron.

Snacks, Cookies, and Cakes

Product	Manufacturer	Serving Size	Calories
FF, Granola Bars, Choc. Flavor Chip	Health Valley	1 bar	140
FF, Granola Bars, Date Almond Flavor	Health Valley	1 bar	140
FF, Granola Bars, Raisin	Health Valley	1 bar	140
FF, Granola Bars, Raspberry	Health Valley	1 bar	140
FF, Granola Bars, Strawberry	Health Valley	1 bar	140
FF, Grissini Style Garlic Bread Sticks	Stella D'oro	3 bread sticks	60
FF, Grissini Style Original Bread Sticks	Stella D'oro	3 bread sticks	60
FF, Holiday Ring	Entenmann's	1 oz.	80
FF, Pineapple Crunch Loaf	Entenmann's	1.3 oz.	90
FF, Potato Chips, Maui Onion	Louise's	1 oz.	100
FF, Potato Chips, Mesquite Barbecue	Louise's	1 oz.	100
FF, Potato Chips, Original	Louise's	1 oz.	100
FF, Potato Chips, Vinegar and Salt	Louise's	1 oz.	100
FF, Premium Cracker Crumbs	Nabisco	2 Tbsp.	50
FF, Premium Saltine Crackers	Nabisco	5 crackers	50
FF, Pretzel Chips	Mr. Phipp's	1 oz.	110
FF, Pretzel Sticks	Mr. Salty	1 oz.	110

Compact, tight leaves indicate the best globe artichokes.
Brown blemishes do not affect quality.

Snacks, Cookies, and Cakes

Product	Manufacturer	Serving Size	Calories
FF, Pretzel Twists	Mr. Salty	1 oz.	110
FF, Raspberry Cheese Buns	Entenmann's	1 bun	50
FF, Raspberry Cheese Pastry	Entenmann's	1.3 oz.	100
Fruit Bars, FF, Bakes, Blueberry Apple	Health Valley	1 bar	90
Fruit Bars, FF, Bakes, Raspberry	Health Valley	1 bar	90
Fruit Bars, FF, Bakes, Strawberry	Health Valley	1 bar	90
Fudge Brownie	Entenmann's	1 brownie	110
Lemon Custard Cake	Betty Crocker	1/2 cake	150
Melba Toast	Lance	2 pieces	30
Oh Berry FF, Strawberry Wafers	Sunshine Biscuit Co.	8 cookies	100
Snacks, Apple Chips	Weight Watchers	3/4 oz.	70
Snackwells, FF, Cinnamon Graham Snacks	Nabisco	1/2 oz.	50
Snackwells, FF, Devil's Food Cookie Cakes	Nabisco	1/2 oz.	50
Snackwells, FF, Wheat Crackers	Nabisco	1/2 oz.	50
Traditional	Betty Crocker	1/2 cake	130

Mature apples have a fruity aroma and brown seeds.
Avoid apples with bruises or other blemishes.

Soups

Product	Manufacturer	Serving Size	Calories
Beef Broth (bouillon)	Campbell's	4 oz.	16
Bouillon Cubes, beef	Steero	1 cube	6
Bouillon Cubes, Chicken	Steero	1 cube	8
Broth, FF, Beef, no salt	Health Valley	6.9 oz.	15
Broth, FF, Chicken	Health Valley	6.9 oz.	20
Broth, FF, Beef, with salt	Health Valley	6.9 oz.	15
Broth, Instant, Beef Flavor	Weight Watchers	1 packet	8
Broth, Instant, Chicken Flavor	Weight Watchers	1 packet	8
Chicken Broth, Healthy Request	Campbell's	8 oz.	16
Chili, FF, mild vegetarian, with black beans	Health Valley	5 oz.	70
Chili, FF, mild vegetarian, w/3 beans	Health Valley	5 oz.	70
Chili, FF, spicy vegetarian, w/black beans	Health Valley	5 oz.	70
Consomme, beef	Campbell's	4 oz.	25
Cup-a-Soup, Chicken broth	Lipton	6 fl. oz.	20
Italian Tomato	Campbell's	4 oz.	90
New England Clam Chowder	Weight Watchers	7.5 oz.	90
Soup Mix, Beefy Onion	Lipton	8 fl. oz.	25

Sweet peppers, whether red or green, should
have a shiny exterior.

Soups

Product	Manufacturer	Serving Size	Calories
Soup Mix, Onion	Lipton	8 fl. oz.	20
Soup Mix, Onion-Mushroom	Lipton	8 fl. oz.	40
Soup Mix, Vegetable	Lipton	8 fl. oz.	40
Split Pea, Soup	Andersen's	7.5 oz.	130

Buy parsley with fresh, crisp, green tops.
They should have little or no bulb formation.

Vegetables

Product	Manufacturer	Serving Size	Calories
Alfalfa seeds, sprouted, raw	generic	1 cup	10
Artichoke hearts, water packed, drained	generic	8 oz. jar	74
Artichokes, globe or french, cooked, drained	generic	1 artichoke	55
Asparagus, canned, spears	generic	4 spears	10
Asparagus, fzn., cooked	generic	4 spears	15
Asparagus, raw, cooked	generic	4 spears	15
Baby Carrots, fresh	generic	1 cup	45
Baby Carrots, frozen	generic	1 cup	55
Bean Sprouts, cooked, drained	generic	1 cup	25
Bean Sprouts, raw	generic	1 cup	30
Bean Dip, Jalapeño flavor	Wise	2 Tbsp.	25
Beans, Snap, canned	generic	1 cup	25
Beans, Snap, frozen, French-style	generic	1 cup	35
Beans, Snap, raw, French-style	generic	1 cup	45
Beet Greens, cooked, drained	generic	1 cup	40
Beets, canned, cooked, diced, sliced	generic	1 cup	55
Beets, cooked, drained, sliced, diced	generic	1 cup	55
Beets, cooked, drained, whole	generic	2 beets	30
Broccoli, fzn., chopped	generic	1 cup	50

The skin of an onion should be very dry.

Vegetables

Product	Manufacturer	Serving Size	Calories
Broccoli, fzn., pieces	generic	1 piece	10
Broccoli, raw, 1/2 inch	generic	1 cup	45
Brussel Sprouts	Green Giant	1/2 cup	40
Brussel Sprouts, frozen	Green Giant	1/2 cup	7
Brussel Sprouts, frozen	Hanover	1/2 cup	40
Butter Beans	Hanover	1/2 cup	80
Butter Beans, in Sauce	Hanover	1/2 cup	100
Butter Beans, tender cooked	S + W	1/2 cup	100
Button Mushrooms	generic	1 cup	20
Cabbage	Dole	1/2 head	18
Cabbage, Chinese, pak-choi, cooked, drained	generic	1 cup	20
Cabbage, common varieties, raw, shredded	generic	1 cup	15
Cabbage, Pe-tsai, raw, pieces,	generic	1 cup	10
Cabbage, red, raw, shredded	generic	1 cup	20
Cabbage, Savoy, raw, shredded	generic	1 cup	20
California Sliced Tomato	Contadina	1/2 cup	40
Carrots, canned, diced	Libby's	1/2 cup	20
Carrots, canned, sliced, drained	generic	1 cup	35

For the best okra, buy the full, tender pods.

Vegetables

Product	Manufacturer	Serving Size	Calories
Carrots, cooked, sliced, drained, fzn.	generic	1 cup	55
Carrots, cooked, sliced, drained, raw	generic	1 cup	70
Carrots, diced	Seneca	1/2 cup	20
Carrots, diced, fancy	S + W	1/2 cup	30
Carrots, julienne, French style, fancy	S + W	1/2 cup	30
Carrots, raw, without crowns and tips, grated	generic	1 cup	45
Carrots, raw, without crowns & tips, whole	generic	1 cup	45
Carrots, sliced	Libby's	1/2 cup	20
Carrots, sliced	Seneca	1/2 cup	20
Carrots, sliced, fancy	S + W	1/2 cup	30
Carrots, sliced, water packed	S + W	1/2 cup	30
Carrots, whole tiny, fancy	S + W	1/2 cup	30
Cauliflower, cooked, drained, frozen	generic	1 cup	35
Cauliflower, cooked, drained, raw	generic	1 cup	30
Cauliflower, raw	generic	1 cup	25
Celery, diced	generic	1 Tbsp.	1.25
Celery, pascal type, raw, diced	generic	1 cup	20
Celery, pascal, raw, large outer stalk	generic	1 stalk	5
Cherry Tomato	generic	1 tomato	6.25
Chervil	generic	1 tsp.	1

Coconuts have a high concentration of saturated fat.

Vegetables

Product	Manufacturer	Serving Size	Calories
Chopped Tomatoes	generic	1 cup	25
Collards, cooked, drained	generic	1 cup	25
Corn	Green Giant	1/2 cup	70
Corn, Frozen White Shoe Peg	Hanover	1/2 cup	80
Corn, Frozen White Sweet	Hanover	1/2 cup	80
Corn, Frozen Yellow Sweet	Hanover	1/2 cup	80
Corn, Golden Vacuum Pack	Libby's	1/2 cup	80
Corn, sweet, cooked, drained, fzn. kernels	generic	1 cup	135
Corn, sweet, cooked, drained	generic	1 ear	60
Corn, White Vacuum Pack	Libby's	1/2 cup	80
Cream Style Corn	Libby's	1/2 cup	80
Eggplant, cooked, steamed	generic	1/2 cup	25
Endive, curley, raw	generic	1 cup	10
FF, Refried Beans	Rosarita	1/2 cup	80
Four Bean Salad	Hanover	1/2 cup	80
Fresh spinach	generic	1/2 cup	12
Frozen stir-fry vegetables	generic	1 lb.	150
Green Beans & Wax Beans	S & W	1/2 cup	20
green beans, canned, unsalted, drained	generic	1 cup	45

Avoid overripe bananas.
Buy only the plump and smooth fruit.

Vegetables

Product	Manufacturer	Serving Size	Calories
Green Beans, cut, frozen	Hanover	1/2 cup	20
Green Beans, cut, canned	Green Giant	1/2 cup	16
Green Beans, cut, canned	Libby's	1/2 cup	20
Green Beans, cut, canned	Owatonna	1/2 cup	20
Green Beans, cut, canned	Seneca	1/2 cup	20
Green Beans, cut, French Natural Pack	Seneca	1/2 cup	20
Green Beans, cut, French Style, Blue Lake	Libby's	1/2 cup	25
Green Beans, cut, French Style, canned	Green Giant	1/2 cup	16
Green Beans, cut, French Style, frozen	Southland	3 oz.	25
Green Beans, cut, frozen	Green Giant	1/2 cup	14
Green Beans, cut, frozen	Southland	3 oz.	25
Green Beans, cut, Natural Pack, canned	Seneca	1/2 cup	20
Green Beans, cut, Premium Blue Lake	S & W	1/2 cup	20
Green Beans, cut Water Pack, canned	S & W	1/2 cup	20
Green Beans, Dilled, canned	S & W	1/2 cup	60
Green Beans, French Premium, Blue Lake	S & W	1/2 cup	20

Bananas are high in potassium.

Vegetables

Product	Manufacturer	Serving Size	Calories
Green Beans, French Style, canned	Libby's	1/2 cup	20
Green Beans, French Style, canned	Owatonna	1/2 cup	20
Green Beans, French Style, canned	Seneca	1/2 cup	20
Green Beans, Harvest Fresh Cut, frozen	Green Giant	1/2 cup	16
Green Beans, Italian Cut, frozen	Hanover	1/2 cup	35
Green Beans, Kitchen Sliced, canned	Green Giant	1/2 cup	16
Green Beans, Whole, Blue Lake, frozen	Hanover	1/2 cup	30
Green Beans, Whole, canned	Libby's	1/2 cup	20
Green Beans, Whole, canned	Seneca	1/2 cup	20
Green Beans, Whole, Fancy, Stringless	S & W	1/2 cup	20
Green Beans, Whole, Vertical Pack, canned	S & W	1/2 cup	20
Green Bell Pepper	generic	1 medium	15
Hot green chili peppers, chopped	generic	4 oz.	17
Italian Style Pear Tomato	Contadina	1/2 cup	25
Italian Style Pear Tomato	S & W	1/2 cup	25
Italian Style Stewed Tomato	Contadina	1/2 cup	35

Look for tomatoes with little or no green core.
They should be firm, but not hard.

Vegetables

Product	Manufacturer	Serving Size	Calories
Italian Style Stewed Tomato	S & W	1/2 cup	35
Kidney Beans, dark red, lite 50% less salt	S & W	1/2 cup	120
Kidney Beans, dark red, canned	Green Giant	1/2 cup	90
Kidney Beans, dark red, canned	Hanover	1/2 cup	110
Kidney Beans, dark red, canned	Trappey's	1/2 cup	90
Kidney Beans, Jalapeno, light red	Trappey's	1/2 cup	90
Kidney Beans, light red	Green Giant	1/2 cup	90
Kidney Beans, light red	Trappey's	1/2 cup	90
Kidney Beans, light red, in sauce	Hanover	1/2 cup	120
Lettuce, raw	generic	1 head	20
Lima Beans	Libby's	1/2 cup	80
Lima Beans, baby, frozen	Hanover	1/2 cup	110
Lima Beans, canned	Seneca	1/2 cup	80
Lima Beans, small, fancy	S & W	1/2 cup	80
Mushrooms, canned	generic	1 cup	35
Mushrooms, raw	generic	1 cup	20
Mustard greens	generic	1 cup	20
New Potatoes	generic	1 potato	58
Onion, purple	generic	1 small	55

Radishes should be firm and crisp with a good shape and color.

Vegetables

Product	Manufacturer	Serving Size	Calories
nion, raw	generic	1 cup	55
arsley, raw	generic	10 sprigs	5
arsnips	generic	1 cup	125
eas, green frozen	generic	1 cup	125
eppers, hot chili, raw	generic	1 pepper	20
eppers, sweet	generic	1 pepper	15
otatoes, cooked, aked, no skin	generic	1 potato	145
otatoes, cooked, aked, with skin	generic	1 potato	220
umpkin, oked, mashed	generic	1 cup	50
adish, raw	generic	1 radish	5
eady Cut eeled Tomato	S & W	1/2 cup	25
ed Bell pepper	generic	1 pepper	15
ed Potatoes	generic	1 potato	80
efried Beans d Green Chili	Little Pancho	1/2 cup	80
uerkraut, canned, lids, liquid	generic	1 cup	45
aweed, raw	generic	1 oz.	10
redded Lettuce	generic	1 Tbsp.	10
ow Peas	generic	1 cup	65
aghetti, raw	generic	2 lb.	138
anish onion	generic	1 cup	55
inach (canned)	Harvest Fresh	1/2 cup	25
inach Fresh Boiled	S & W	1/2 cup	21
inach, Chopped or ole Leaf (canned)	Del Monte	1/2 cup	25

Ale refers to a lightly colored beer.

Vegetables

Product	Manufacturer	Serving Size	Calories
Spinach, frozen	Green Giant	1/2 cup	25
Spinach, Premium Northwest (canned)	S & W	1/2 cup	25
Spinach, raw, chopped	generic	1 cup	10
Stewed Tomato	Contadina	1/2 cup	35
Stewed Tomato	Del Monte	1/2 cup	35
Stewed Tomato	Hunt's	1/2 cup	35
Stewed Tomato	S & W	1/2 cup	35
Stewed Tomato, 50% less salt	S & W	1/2 cup	35
Stewed Tomato, Mexican Style	S & W	1/2 cup	40
Sun dried Tomatoes	generic	1 tomato	25
Sweet Potatoes, cooked, boiled, w/o skin	generic	1 potato	160
Tomato, green	generic	1 tomato	30
Tomato, red	generic	1 tomato	24
Turnips	generic	1 cup	30
Water Chestnuts, canned	generic	1 cup	70
Water Pack	S & W	1/2 cup	90
Watercress	generic	1/2 cup	2
Wedges, Tomato	Del Monte	1/2 cup	30
Whole Peeled Tomato	Contadina	1/2 cup	25
Whole Peeled Tomato	Del Monte	1/2 cup	25
Whole Peeled Tomato	S & W	1/2 cup	25
Whole Tomato	Hunt's	1/2 cup	20
Yellow Beans	generic	1 cup	45
Yellow Bell Pepper	generic	1 medium	15

Bean sprouts grow from mung beans, and are harvested and sold within six days from the time they first appear.

Notes

....

....

....

....

....

....

....

....

....

....

....

....

Notes

**Fat Free Foods
Mail Order Catalogue**

For More Information,
please print your name and address
on the form below and mail to:

Onomy House Publishing
Post Office Box 1151
Alpharetta, Georgia 30239

Name _____

Address _____

_____

City _____

State _____ Zip Code _____

Country _____ – Thank You!

Quantity discounts are available
on bulk purchases of this book
for educational, business,
or sales promotions use.

For information, please write to:
Sales Department,
Onomy House Publishing
Post Office Box 1151
Alpharetta, Georgia 30239